...Learning to Dance in the Rain

A Parent's Guide to Neuroblastoma Diagnosis, Treatment and Beyond

Rachel A. Ormsby

Learning to Dance in the Rain. A Parent's Guide to Neuroblastoma Diagnosis, Treatment and Beyond

DancingintherainNB is part of MJ Ministries Inc. a qualified IRS Section 501(c) (3) Organization.

ISBN-13: 978-0989427739 (DancingintherainNB)

ISBN-10: 0989427730

Printed in the United States of America

DEDICATION

This book is dedicated to our children Nathan and Kate because childhood cancer affects all the children in a family.

ACKNOWLEDGEMENTS

Thank you to my husband Scott for convincing me to take on this project and supporting me through it.

Thank you to the friends and family who have proof read each version of this book to make it better.

Thank you to Dr. Sonata Jodele for being the technical advisor for this book.

PREFACE

When Nathan was first diagnosed with neuroblastoma in 2006, our family entered a world we knew nothing about. The world of childhood cancer is terrifying and complicated. We had a lot to learn and quickly. We had to learn about treatments, scans, blood draws, labs, medicines, and side effects, including how to handle them. We looked for help from other parents and Nathan's medical staff. One thing that would have helped was a guide that we could have read and made notes in as we traveled this path. A guide to all those things other families have already learned. Something we could have carried around with us that would help us make sense of this new vocabulary and the things we needed to know. This book is for just that purpose. It is intended to help navigate some of the things you will find during your child's treatment and recovery from cancer. It is not intended to be inclusive or to replace the doctors; it is intended to share experiences and knowledge, parent to parent. This book contains what my family has learned from the medical staffs we have worked with, other parents, and the kids we have been privileged to meet on our journey.

This book is organized into sections by topic. The order of the topics is loosely the order you may see things in your journey. They are not in order of priority.

The first two sections are "The Beginning" and "Diagnosis." They discuss our family's experiences through the diagnosis phase of childhood cancer. It describes how we learned something was wrong with Nathan and what we did after getting this information. These sections give an introduction to our family.

"Cancer 101" is intended to be a short course on cancer treatments and scans. It contains a summary of treatments that will most likely be in a child's fight with neuroblastoma. Each area describes what treatments are like and what the purpose of each is. Then there is a little bit about our experience and the things we learned during that time. This section also includes an introduction to each of the scans and tests that are used during diagnosis and treatment. Many of these scans have things you as a parent can do to help your child get through the scan, and, potentially, receive a more accurate result. There is a LOT of information out there about treatments and scans. The intent is to identify the important parts from a parent's perspective. In the end it is up to you to talk to your medical team to fill in the details to get a complete picture.

"Bone Marrow Transplant" describes the unique things that are associated with a bone marrow transplant (BMT). This section is separate from the other treatment sections since it is such a large and unique treatment. There are many things that apply specifically to BMT.

"How to Manage Cancer 101" is about my family's experiences and the things we have learned during our journey. There are topics like assigning blame, keeping family and friends informed, loving on the other family members, accepting help, defining primary and alternate care givers, and relating those funny hospital humor stories. We have met a lot of people through this journey; many have helped us cope and taught us how to get through it.

"Types of Medicine" is about the many types of treatments and medicines available. This section talks about things like clinical trials, FDA approved drugs, supplements, and researching new medicine or treatment options. With all the information out there, we found that the world of cancer drugs can be confusing. When fighting cancer there is a whole new world you may never have thought about or realized is available for you and your child. Again, this section is not meant to be inclusive; treatment options change as advances are made.

"Long Term Side Effects" is about the late effects that Nathan has experienced and how we have addressed them. Inevitably, on the road to recovery some long term side effects or late effects, start showing up. There is a lot of documentation out there on what these effects are. We have found little on how to handle them other than "just tough it out". This approach was just not good enough. We, as a family, spent a lot of time successfully helping Nathan work through many of these, finding new ways for his brain to learn and grow. We hope it gives you and your child a starting point in handling these areas.

"Wish Trip" describes the trip Nathan was given by the Special Wish Foundation. When Nathan was offered a "Wish" we knew very little about them or how they were awarded, etc. This section describes our trip so that when the time comes for your "Wish" from your local "Wish" foundation you can have an example of what one is like. It was a phenomenal, loving, once in a lifetime experience. While reading this section you can make notes for your future family vacation.

"Organization and Resources" is a short list of those groups that helped us. There are a seemingly unlimited number of organizations and resources out there to help families. Many of these groups we found by word of mouth from other parents. This section briefly describes some of them and how they helped us. Each entry has contact information for the organization.

Finally, there is a glossary of terms and acronyms. The field of medicine has its own language. Eventually all of these phrases and words will be clear to you. Until then, this list can help translate what they are talking about.

CONTENTS

CHAPTER 1. THE BEGINNING

This story is about my family's ongoing battle with childhood cancer. My son, Nathan was diagnosed with stage 4 neuroblastoma at 3 ½ years old and is still fighting it at age 10. Our path has taken us to 5 main hospitals, through many rounds of chemotherapy and many alternative forms of treatment that are now main stream, and led us to meet many, many, many amazing adults and children. The goal of this text is to give parents an overview of what is to come and things that can help them through the battle of childhood cancer. This is written from our family's perspective and is not meant to cover every possibility, treatment, doctor's opinions or outcome. It is meant to give some direction and guidance via learning experiences and people we have met along our way. It will show the trials and heartache we went through but will also show some things that we did well that made life easier and what we now know we should have done to make other things better. It is our hope that by sharing our experiences of Nathan's journey that we may help another child and their parents along their path.

November 12 was the day Nathan was born. There was no question in my mind that our Happily Ever After was about to start. My husband Scott and I had spent 7 long years trying to have him, and he was finally here. We felt that all the trials and tribulations of our early years of marriage were now over. We eloped right after we got engaged. The first year of our marriage we spent mostly apart as Scott went to Air Force pilot training in Texas while I stayed in Virginia to work and keep my engineering career going. Eighteen months later, we moved to Northern California where Scott flew C-5s and I worked as a NASA contractor. This meant weeks and sometimes months apart while he flew around the world and I traveled for my job. After a few years of this we decided it was finally time to have children. Our careers were solid and so was our marriage. It turned out that for us this was not to be as easy as we expected. After years of trying to have Nathan, we found out that I was unable to have children on my own. We spent the next 5 years in fertility treatment of one sort or another. None of our efforts were working, but we had one very last chance to have kids of our own through in vitro fertilization before we would attempt to adopt our children. That one last chance worked, against all odds. We found out I was pregnant, and now here he was.

Nathan's first couple years were delightful. He's a smart little boy with a wonderfully upbeat personality. He was not a complainer and in general just wanted to have fun. He was outgoing and did not require us to be on hand with him constantly. When he was 20 months old and we went to the Air Force Ball, his babysitter, Kyle, arrived at the door. Nathan ran to the door, opened it, smiled at Kyle, turned to me and said "Mommy, you need to leave." That is a well-adjusted little boy.

My pregnancy with Nathan had been filled with one complication after another. We decided that having more children would be very dangerous for me. The worst complications happened during child birth and I almost did not survive. We proceeded with adoption plans for our second child. Nathan's sister, Kate, arrived when Nathan was 2 ½ years old. What a bright bundle of joy she was. Our family was now complete. Nathan completely adored his sister and rarely left her side. They shared a room and he would frequently just watch her sleep. Kate was his favorite person.

The year started out as great year for our family. It started with one of the happiest days of our lives, the finalization of Kate's adoption. She was ours forever. A bit later Scott was promoted to Lieutenant Colonel in the Air Force. We found our home and settled in. Our church home was wonderful where we were welcomed with open arms. I had found a bible study group for moms where I had women to learn from and share with. Life was going so well Scott and I took a great vacation in Paris, just the two of us, no kids. Unfortunately, when we returned home, things changed.

Just after Kate's first birthday in July, Nathan started having pain in his right shin. We had just had the shin and leg examined less than a month before, but the doctor and X-rays found nothing. Then, Nathan started a high fever. After three days with an unexplained fever the mom books say to take him to the doctors. I was not really worried about him because Kate also had a fever; in my mind they had the same ear infection or bug. The Air Force base pediatric clinic where we were stationed did not have an appointment for us that day, but they were uncomfortable leaving the fever for the next day when they did have an appointment available. They recommended we go to the Emergency Room. The Air Force hospital staff was fantastic. They immediately diagnosed Kate with an ear infection, gave her antibiotics and turned their attention to Nathan. Nathan did not have an ear infection, his ears were clear. *Ok, then what?* They started to ask for other symptoms. *Could his leg pain be related?* Then the series of doctors started coming one after another as they tried to figure out which specialty would be best to diagnose his problem. We ended with Orthopedics. This doctor was amazing, straight and to the point. *"You will go to the Children's Hospital; they will put a needle in Nathan's right hip and take out a sample of the inflammation for testing. We will then find out what kind of infection is causing the fever and swelling in his right leg".* We learned that day that shin pain can mean inflammation in the hip. The doctor also recommended that we find a place for Kate to spend the night and pack a bag for Nathan and myself in case they kept us overnight. I felt a little nervous at this point, could there really be something wrong with my little boy?

The potential for an overnight hospital stay may seem like a very straight forward request. However, there was a problem. Scott was on a month long trip for the Air Force, and could not come home. Worst of all, it was tough to get hold of him on the phone most days. I was going to have to deal with this without him for now. I kept saying to myself that it is just something minor. I can do this for just one night. We found a bed for Kate at a friend's house, I got Nathan's and my bag packed, and off we went to the children's hospital. It is funny the details you remember in a crisis and the details you forget. I remembered our toothbrushes, I remember clothes and Nathan's stuffed animal, but I forgot to get directions to the hospital and I did not have a GPS or smart phone. Nathan really enjoyed this part of the trip, being in the back seat and chastising me that I was going to get him lost. We finally found the hospital, found parking, found the Emergency Department (ED), and checked in. It is interesting to look now back at this first impression of our home for the next 10 months, the smell, the people, the hallways that I would eventually figure out, the pictures of the children hanging up of whom Nathan would eventually be one, the first impressions of the staff and more.

The ED staff was friendly enough. Nathan and I were sent right back to a room since the Air Force doctor had called ahead and let them know about our situation. But, when we saw the orthopedic resident, they were less than impressed with our situation. I got the feeling he was thinking I was an over protective mom that was blowing things a bit out of proportion. After a brief examination we saw the orthopedic surgeon who confirmed the resident's suspicion that Nathan has some minor inflammation in his hip and a stronger anti-inflammatory medicine would fix him up. *Oh good,* I felt, but was not quite sure they got it. They told us they would give Nathan medicine that would knock out the inflammation and we could go home the next day. Here was the start of the internal battle I would have throughout treatment. I wanted to respect the doctor's opinion and expertise but sometimes I had a difference of opinion. When was it correct to speak out and when was it correct to do as instructed? Should I mention the needle the Air Force doctor had discussed? I have found that in general it is always a good idea to discuss your concerns with the doctors so that in the end you can completely understand their instructions.

When looking back at this ED visit I can now see some of the doctor's point of view of Nathan's presentation. Here was a 3 year old boy that was happy and upbeat. He was not really showing any discomfort unless you touched the hip or he had to put his full weight on it. He did have a fever but was not acting sick. And, really, the number of orthopedic patients in the ED that are diagnosed with cancer is miniscule. To give this resident credit, when he found out that there was something wrong with Nathan and he had missed it, he visited us every day while he was there just to chat and see how things were going. I really appreciated that.

Nathan and I spent the night in the Almost Home Unit at the children's hospital, where children stay that will be at the hospital less than 24 hours. The staff was simply wonderful. They got us settled down and the staff spoiled that boy rotten. He had a great time. The medicine did make him feel better. He was smiling, his fever was down and he was walking around a bit better, not to mention he was putting his considerable charm on the nurses and staff. The next morning the orthopedic doctor and his residents came by on rounds and declared Nathan cured. *Oh, that was not right.* Nope, I felt they did not get this, but do I say something? Yup, I sure do. *"Excuse me, but I don't think you got this. I don't think the medicine did as you described. Tylenol worked just as well. I think there is more to this."* I heard myself telling them. I really don't think they appreciated my candidness. I received a very polite response on how I should go home, give him 3 to 5 days (with no additional medicine) and if everything is not better, give the orthopedic doctor a call to come in for an appointment. *Right. Ok. It is not going to happen that way.*

I departed the hospital with a very bad feeling that we had missed something, picked up Kate and went home, and talked to Scott on the phone and relayed my concerns. We both agreed there was more to this and we needed to pursue it. It took about an hour before I was back on the phone with the Pediatrics Clinic on the Air Force base to request another appointment the next day. When Nathan crawled to the bathroom in the middle of the night, fear and foreboding started taking a serious hold on me. When we arrived at the clinic the Air Force Major that greeted us was over the top friendly and helpful. I briefly gave her our story and she was on the phone with the orthopedic surgeon from the children's hospital. I did not hear all the conversation but heard just enough to know when I saw him that afternoon he was not going to be happy to see us.

This time we were treated differently, this time Nathan was sick and there was something they had to find out. This time the staff was very kind and tender to both of us. This time the bag was packed for a week, not overnight, and I knew how to get to the hospital. After Nathan's exam we were informed they were going to do an ultrasound of his right hip. This was our first taste of scans and technicians. Radiology technicians still are some of our favorite people; they really know how to spoil a child to get them to sit still for a scan. Nathan was put under anesthesia for his ultrasound since he was so small and in so much pain. How horrifying. While getting him ready we giggled, smiled, joked, and played games until it was time. When he went back to get his scan I started another tradition of pacing a deep groove into the hospital floor. When he came out I will NEVER forget the look on the faces of the doctor (anesthesiologist) and technicians. The scan showed something was wrong. I was told by the doctor present that the scan came back positive. No one knew what it was positive for, but we all knew that things were about to change for us for good.

Now I had to do something I had not done in the past 15 years of marriage, I needed to bring Scott home from his Air Force assignment. All of the problems and logistics of doing this did not even come to my mind. The Air Force would need to find a replacement test pilot for Scott on no notice; his supervisor would need to completely back him to get him home. I did not expect that he would even be able to come home immediately, but I needed to tell him. I walked out the front of the hospital and called Scott. *"You need to come home now; something is wrong with Nathan."*

CHAPTER 2. DIAGNOSIS

Our summer and our lives had suddenly completely changed. The Air Force and Scott's coworkers made it possible for Scott to come home from his trip. Kate was wondering where mom had gone, and now we had to find out what the first scan showed. What was the "something wrong" they had seen on the scan? We spent the next couple weeks in the hospital while the doctors figured it out. Nathan bounced around the floors until that very memorable day when the oncologist came in, introduced himself and told us we were moving to the Hematology/Oncology (Hem/Onc) floor. I have to admit, I knew absolutely nothing about Hematology or Oncology and more importantly did not really want to. Nathan had not been diagnosed yet, but according to the doctor, there really wasn't any other option other than some form of cancer, but for some reason they were careful to not use that word.

Over the previous couple weeks what started as shin pain and a fever of 102 F had turned into something horrible. Nathan arrived at the hospital with a simple limp. It did not slow him down; he ran the halls, visited, played the balloon drums, and had us wheel him to all the different aquariums in the hospital so he could visit the fish; we had to see how big the baby fish were getting. A couple weeks later, the boy could not walk. His fever was uncontrollable with medicine, he was completely pale and would only play the balloon drums if they were tied to his bed and low enough he could reach them without lifting his arms. He still enjoyed visiting the fish, but would only lay there and look at the fish without talking to them. I still cannot imagine how close we came to losing him.

Then our new lives started when Nathan was finally diagnosed. Diagnosis date is a set of numbers that I will never forget 8/8/06, two days after my own birthday. The pathology report came back positive for neuroblastoma. I remember the conversation with his primary oncologist clearly, "It is not a straight forward leukemia like we had hoped, it is neuroblastoma". How horrible could this disease be if leukemia was "straight forward" when compared to it. Now we needed to get busy. There were many scans to perform to show the doctors

Nathan's "Bad Guys" as we would call them. I remember nothing moving fast enough. *When were we going to start fighting back against this disease that was killing my son?*

First they had to run a bone scan, MIBG scan, CT scan, GFR, bone marrow aspirations, MRI, and I'm sure more I cannot remember. Then we had to wait to see what stage they assigned to his disease so that we could determine what treatment plan he should follow. Then he had surgery to put in a central line into the big vessel close to the heart and they took out whatever disease they could that was located on and near his left adrenal gland. Then we had to wait for his recovery from surgery so that he was healthy enough to dump chemotherapy into him. It was all very slow. I have heard people say over and over again that you should pay attention when your children are small because in a blink of an eye they will be grown. I have to say I blinked my eyes over and over again and still life moved slower and slower. Every scan, every treatment, every moment, took an eternity. I kept thinking to myself, one more blink and the cancer will be gone. One more blink and Nathan will be grown with kids of his own and this slow nightmare will be over.

CHAPTER 3. CANCER 101

During the first week after Nathan's diagnosis Scott and I sat down with Nathan's doctor to have our Cancer 101 speech. Apparently parents only retain about 10 percent of these types of conversations. If we only remembered 10 percent, I'm really happy to have forgotten the other 90 percent. This is the first time Nathan's issue got a name: Cancer. In this talk we learned why cancer was bad and that the body did not fight it because the body did not see the cancer as foreign. We learned that remission was having less than a certain number of cancer cells in the body and that it really did not apply to this form of cancer. Neuroblastoma was so bad you either got completely rid of it, or you kept trying until you did. We learned that for neuroblastoma they would be talking in terms of "complete response" or "no evidence of disease" (no disease can be seen by scans or biopsies), "partial response" (the disease level or burden has been reduced by half), or progression (where the disease is growing despite being on therapy). We learned all the different types of blood cells and which ones we cared about and when. We learned the cycle of his chemotherapy, when Nathan would feel fine and when we needed to be extra careful.

Then we asked about prognosis. *What was Nathan's prognosis?* This I can remember very clearly. "Every patient is different. We would need to see how the medicine affected Nathan's disease." What we did know was that with Nathan's age of over 30 months and the extent his disease had spread through his body, Nathan had "high risk metastatic disease". Metastatic disease is where the cancer has spread from the primary tumor to other parts of the body. In Nathan's case it had spread from the left adrenal gland to most of his bones.

An important thing we learned that week was that Scott and I were allowed to ask as many questions as we would like. We were also allowed to ask the same question over and over again as many times as we needed. We could have doctors and nurses write in our journal the things that we did not understand. We were allowed to cry. We were allowed to laugh and spoil this boy as rotten as we could. We were allowed to ask for help at any time from anyone who would give it. We also learned that even if you do not ask for help, it will still be given in great quantities.

We learned that there is a limit to the amount of medicine a child can be given. We learned what an allergic or paradoxical reaction (having the opposite effect) to a drug looked like. Nathan had been in the hospital for weeks, and he had been on pain medicine the entire time. The dose had been increased to help him with his additional pain. Nathan started having bad muscle spasms; we think from all the pain medicine. He could not sleep, and he could not get comfortable. The resident gave him a sedative medicine to help calm him down and let him get some sleep. Unfortunately Nathan had the opposite reaction to the sedative. He was hallucinating about bugs on the wall, he saw shadows coming at him, and he was just shaking all over. I had to bear hug him for four hours as the drug wore off. Otherwise, he surely would have hurt himself. Now whenever asked if Nathan has a medicine allergy, we say yes to the sedative. It may not be exactly an allergy, but we definitely do not want him to get it again.

During these first couple weeks after diagnosis we found that kids are best treated at a children's hospital. The hospital staff knows how to handle little kids that do not feel well. They know how to calm a child and distract him or her from something unpleasant. They know that kids still need to be kids even when sick. They know how valuable the parents are and treat them very gingerly.

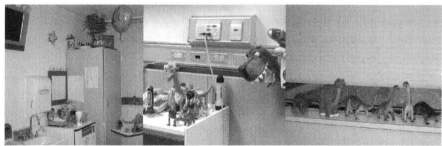

Figure 1 Nathan's First Oncology Hospital Room

We were able to decorate Nathan's hospital rooms with as many dinosaurs that we could fit into them. Nathan LOVED dinosaurs and everyone knew it. We had dinosaurs arriving in the room at all times.

We had puppets to make battles, and we had hard plastic dinosaurs, soft fluffy dinosaurs, dinosaur balloons, and so on. We had every dinosaur imaginable to help make this little boy happy. If you did visit, you had to be prepared to do dinosaur battle.

We learned how truly big Nathan's heart is. Before the surgery to remove the primary tumor, his grandparents wanted to visit him in his room. Nathan would NOT allow them into the room with him. *NO! They cannot come in!* It took a while but we were finally able to find out that our boy was worried that he would give his grandparents whatever bad guys he had and he did not want to get them sick. Parents were apparently immune to bad guys or we were allowed to get them; he never clarified. We explained to him that his bad guys were only in him and it was not possible for him to give them to anyone else. His stress level decreased significantly on that day.

We learned so many more things through our months and years on this new path our lives had taken. The following sections contain some of these things. It is our hope that contained somewhere in these pages there is something that can help make another child and family's journey even a little bit easier.

Journaling

The single most useful thing to us during Nathan's journey was keeping a journal. We started writing a journal shortly after Nathan was admitted to the hospital the first time. It started as me writing notes to tell to Scott things and Scott writing notes back. That quickly turned into a small journaling book that we got at the gift shop. We carried the journal around wherever Nathan went. It was in the hospital room with him, it went to scans with him, and we left it on the kitchen counter when at home. Visitors to the hospital or home would write notes and prayers or tell stories or jokes. We quickly became very dependent on it. We left notes to each other to pass off caretaking each night. It included the events of the day, when his next Tylenol or Benadryl doses were, what concerns we had, things for the other to keep an eye on, funny stories, medicine changes - anything that the other parent would need was written down in the journal. We included questions for the doctors, information on transfusions and reactions, and any episode we needed to relate or track. It is easy to forget things when talking to the doctors. Having it written down gave us a starting point. In the last few pages we kept a running list of Nathan's medicines with dose and frequency.

The journal was important for scans. When a child is getting a scan the technicians are not allowed to discuss the scan with you. They cannot make diagnoses or interpret the scan at all, which is the radiologist's job. However, you as a parent are allowed to sketch what you see. I put the sketches in our journal and then would be able to talk to Scott or the doctors more accurately. Scott would do the same thing for me. When we received the radiologist report, we would make notes on the picture as to what each item meant. Our biggest fear was and still is progression. Any new spot would have severe consequences. It made us feel more comfortable going into a scan knowing where the hot spots had been the last time so at least with an untrained eye we may be able to detect new ones and be prepared when we spoke with the doctor. It was not our responsibility to read a scan, but waiting for the results was always

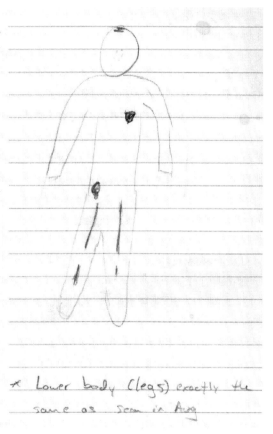

✗ Lower body (legs) exactly the same as Scan in Aug

Figure 2 Sample of Journal Artwork

the hardest thing. Being able to see the scans ourselves helped us prepare for what might be on the radiologist's report.

As part of our Journal we also always had "The List". The list had all the items we wanted to discuss with the doctor. It had questions, like *"When should he get a flu shot?"*, *"Can he go outside?"* and other easy things like that. Sometimes it was harder questions about when to remove his port, what treatment options were available, or anything else we wanted to talk about. We would create this list between doctor appointments. The journal and the list would go with whoever took Nathan in for the appointment. This way all our concerns were answered independent of who went to the doctors. Before "The List" we ALWAYS forgot something and would have to call back or email or just go without for another week. After a while the list was expected. Many times when talking to the doctor, they would ask one of us for the list. Those days we must have looked VERY tired.

Things We Put in Our Journal

- We taped all business cards we felt were important to the inside cover.
- We taped photos throughout the book.
- The List
- The last couple pages were for medicines with doses.
- Visitors signed the book with prayers and well wishes for Nathan and the family.
- Questions for and answers from doctors
- Sketches of scan results
- Funny stories that happened throughout the day
- Anything the doctors or nurses said that we wanted to share with the other parent.
- Described adverse drug reactions
- Anything else we wanted to write down

Sample Journal Entry

15 August

Doctor will be coming by later to help get Nathan to move. The doctor said if we can get him to move around, walk, play, sit up, anything, his bowels will recover from surgery quicker and the sooner he can start chemo.

We need to get a chemo toothbrush and toothpaste

If we saran wrap his incision we can bathe him. Press-n-Seal is recommended. Doctor thinks it is a good idea. Again motion is essential.

Last night we had a great time playing with Andrea and Elena. We opened the new dinosaur and had a blast knocking over the tower. Lots of laughs, smiles, dimples and sheer joy. It was great. We spent a bit of time shooting rocks at Nurse Kelly.

Happy Birthday Grandma Hart

Going to try Phenergan for nausea when needed

On an easier chemo today, should not be as bad.

0845 Dr Ch – ok to get tummy wet. Nurses will help bathe.

1100 Bath, walk to and from nurse's station. Rosalyn helped!

During this journey you receive many pieces of paper. There are lab results, test reports, treatment plans, instructions, etc. We found it best to keep these items in a three ring binder. The binder got larger over time and became more organized with tabs for different topics. The advantage of the binder was we always knew where to put the paper when we got it. More importantly we knew where to find it again later. This may seem simple enough, but when you realize the quantity of paper and the large number of sources of paper, this can be a huge time saver.

Routine

Our family was having a tough time adjusting to our new reality. Everything was new and out of place in our lives. In order to get some sort of control and sanity back we tried to find some form of routine to follow. We had to address Nathan's trips to the hospital for treatment and those visits for fever. We also had to address Scott's work and figure out Kate's care. Additionally, we thought it would be very nice if we could find a way for both parents to get some sleep somewhere, sometime. This is a lot to juggle when your primary focus is on how to care for your sick child. Scott and I finally found a routine that worked for us. Kate had started to attend a childcare center and Scott was back at work. Those days that Nathan was at the hospital, Scott would come to the hospital in the evening with Kate. We would have a moment or two to chat and then I would take Kate home so Scott could take care of Nathan through the night. The next morning Kate and I would arrive back at the hospital to swap back again. Scott would take Kate to daycare and I would be with Nathan that day and through the night. The next night we would repeat this cycle. Scott stayed at the hospital 12 hours followed by me being at the hospital for 36 hours. This routine could go on for weeks depending how long Nathan was in treatment or recovering from a fever. This routine helped define our responsibilities and gave us some idea of a normal for this stage of life. Finding a routine in all the madness allowed us to get rid of the chaos feeling a bit. We felt we could control a little bit of our life if we started with a plan. The plan did not always work but at least we had a starting point. Every family's routine will be different. Try to find one that works for you and then do not be discouraged if it changes frequently.

Hospital Room

We found that we tended to get into a routine in the hospital room itself. When Nathan was admitted, there was a series of things we did each time. Nathan would start by climbing on everything to see what was most comfortable. He would then ignore the resident doctor as best he could. Scott or I would discuss with the staff all the other things that needed to be completed before our stay. We did our admitting paperwork. We went over the current medicine list, when he had the last of each of his medicines, the issues Nathan was having at home, new symptoms, etc. Most of these were written down in the journal. The nurses and doctors would get the "orders", or instructions, in for Nathan's medicines. With the paperwork completed Nathan would have fluids connected and we would settle in.

Once there Scott and I were usually concerned about just a few of the medications and when they could be given next. Not chemotherapy or other fancy medications, but the four that made Nathan feel better, nausea medication, Tylenol, Benadryl, and pain medicine. We used the white board in the room to track them. Most hospital rooms have a white board. The nurses put their names on it and give you other information you may need. We used a small corner of it to write down the times of the next dose of each of these four medications. That way we knew he was given his last dose and how long we had until he could have more. Most nurses would fill it out for us, others did not. Either way, we had the most important information we needed to make Nathan feel better.

Stages of Disease

There are many possible treatment plans and potential treatment options that all depend on how your child's disease is behaving. For example, if the disease has spread from the primary tumor location to other parts of the body, it is necessary to fight that disease aggressively with very strong medicine. However, if the disease is just starting and it has not spread at all, then it would be prudent to not harm the child with more medicine than is needed. To determine the appropriate treatment protocol, the doctors "stage" the disease into manageable groups. Each group or stage has a different treatment protocol. The less severe the stage of the disease the "easier" the treatment can be. The higher the stage or "risk", the more aggressive the disease is and therefore the more aggressive the treatment needs to be.

Here is a basic list of neuroblastoma stages:

Stage 1   the tumor is in one area and can be removed completely by surgery.

Stage 2   the tumor is in one area and may not be able to be removed completely by surgery.

Stage 3   the tumor has grown past the midline of the body from one side to the other.

Stage 4   the disease has spread to other parts of the body

Stage 4s   child is younger than 1 yr old with other more specific criteria

Staging of neuroblastoma can be very complex, many factors are included such as histology (cellular level makeup of the tumor), location of tumor, extent of disease, age of child, etc. Nathan was diagnosed with stage 4 high risk neuroblastoma based on a few factors. One was age; children diagnosed over a certain age are automatically high risk or stage 4. Another was location; the disease had spread throughout his skeleton.

After the disease is staged, the treatment protocol is assigned and treatment can begin. The following sections go through the types of treatments that Nathan received.

Frontline Therapy

The most accepted treatment protocol to fight a child's cancer is called frontline therapy. Frontline therapy is the name for the first series of treatments. It consists of the best, most proven therapies for your child's cancer type and stage. It is frontline therapy that gives your child the best chances to beat the cancer. It is important to discuss the treatment plan and options, if there are any, with your child's doctor. The doctors know the history of the treatment options, the expected side effects, and whether treatment can happen at your home or in the hospital, etc. I repeat again that talking with your child's doctor is always your best first step to understanding what is going to happen as well as to resolve any issues that may come up during treatment.

The frontline therapy protocol for neuroblastoma has various types of treatment possibilities such as surgery, chemotherapy, and radiation. The treatments are put together in an order that has been proven over the years to give the best chance to rid your child of the disease. Each child's disease reacts differently to the treatments, so the best approach is a variety of treatment types. Listed below are the treatments that Nathan had during his journey. Again, each child's disease is different from every other child's disease and must be treated uniquely. Each of the treatments listed will be discussed in greater detail in the sections that follow.

Nathan's protocol specified the following:

- Remove primary tumor – surgery to take out as much disease as possible.
- Two rounds of chemotherapy
- Peripheral stem cell harvest – procedure to take stem cells out of the blood to be used later to recover from bone marrow transplant
- Four more rounds of chemotherapy
- Bone marrow transplant – intense chemotherapy that wipes out bone marrow. Stem cells are given back to restart bone marrow.
- Radiation – radiation to primary tumor bed and other areas of concern
- Cis Retinoic Acid – an oral drug that helps keep the residual neuroblastoma cells from maturing or help them become not cancerous

Nathan's treatment plan did not quite follow this path. As he went through treatment; we needed to make changes to the plan. His cancer was so wide-spread in his bones that the standard frontline therapy did not completely remove his disease. With the help of the doctors, we changed his treatment path a few times. Nathan also received the following treatments (again, each of these items will be discussed in detail in the sections that follow):

- MIBG therapy – radioactive dye treatment. Only available at a few hospitals

- Antibody therapy – antibodies attach to neuroblastoma cells, so the child's immune system can recognize them as foreign (bad) and kill them
- ABT-751 - an experimental drug to prevent progression of disease
- Many more rounds of different types of chemotherapy and additional antibodies

Frontline therapy in many children can clear the bone marrow of disease and clear the rest of the detectable disease from your child. However, it can happen that frontline therapy works somewhat but not enough to proceed onto the next step. Some protocol steps have criteria for proceeding, such as "clear bone marrow", or "minimal residual disease", etc. These criteria are there to help your child. It would be unfortunate to start an aggressive treatment like bone marrow transplant if it has little chance of success. It could leave your child weak and defenseless. If your child is like Nathan and frontline therapy worked wonders but was still not enough, there are secondary options to pursue such as those listed above. The doctors and the neuroblastoma community are always learning and making advances in treatment. Many of Nathan's secondary options, such as MIBG therapy, antibody therapy, and some of the chemotherapy drugs, are now part of frontline therapy.

The sections that follow review each of the options listed above, generally in the order we followed them. The intention here is to give you some idea of each step and the things we learned that helped us get through them. It is not intended to give you an all-inclusive detailed analysis of each treatment option. When Nathan started treatment, we found the amount of information available overwhelming and complex. What we wanted was an overview of what to expect and the terminology we would need to understand so we could find out more detailed information as we needed it. What we found were many sources of detailed information for each of the steps. We had to figure out what we could or could not use as we went along. Once again, discuss all the treatments and concerns with your child's doctor to find their best recommendations.

Removal of Primary Tumor

The best way to kill cancer is to remove it from the body. The cancer cannot grow if it is not in your child's body. There are different times during the course of treatment when the primary tumor can be removed. On occasion, the doctors are able to remove the primary tumor before chemotherapy is started. Other times the tumor is too big and your child needs to wait and let the chemotherapy drugs shrink it enough so the entire tumor can be removed. Sometimes the tumor is twisted around internal organs, the spine, or other areas that are not prudent to go near in surgery.

In cases of metastatic neuroblastoma, initial surgery is often dedicated to get enough tumor for a detailed diagnosis. This procedure is often combined with the central line placement (plastic tube in the big vessel next to the heart used for blood draws and to administer medications). After five (or so) rounds of chemotherapy the tumor should be smaller and harder and, therefore, easier to remove. The child may then have a "second look" surgery to remove the primary tumor and any other disease that can be removed.

Regardless of the stage of your child's disease, taking the tumor out is just the beginning of treatment. Many rounds of chemotherapy are still needed to remove the remaining disease. There are cells, which cannot be detected, floating in your child's system that need to be treated with chemotherapy.

The time finally came to have the surgery to remove Nathan's primary tumor and put a Broviac catheter in place. A Broviac catheter is a central line that leaves the two tubes extruding from the skin. Our son was now going to have 2 tubes sticking out of his chest for what turned out to be over a year. Scott and I spent surgery in the waiting room with family from out of town and friends from church. Our surgeon stopped by after the surgery to inform us that taking out the tumor "couldn't have been easier". The tumor was in one piece and had not wrapped itself around any of Nathan's organs. He was able to remove the entire primary tumor, the left adrenal gland and put the Broviac line in place. Now at least part of Nathan's bad guys were gone, never to return, but there was a lot of metastatic disease in his bones to be treated.

Chemotherapy

The main attack against cancer is chemotherapy. Chemotherapy drugs work by killing rapidly reproducing cells throughout the body. These include things like hair cells, which makes the hair fall out, blood cells and so on. Each chemotherapy drug attacks specific types of cells; therefore, to get maximum effectiveness, the doctors prescribe a "cocktail" of drugs that work together. Chemotherapy is very caustic and strenuous on the body. Children are much stronger than adults when it comes to recovering from treatment and get relatively large doses for their body surface area. Doctors use body surface area to calculate the amount of medicine to give a child.

It is very hard to describe what your child will go through, and every child will react a bit differently. You cannot prevent many of the side effects no matter how hard you try or how much you want to. You can, however, spend your time trying to keep track of the things that work on your child. I recommend keeping a list of the chemotherapy drugs your child receives in the back of your journal with the specific side effects they cause. If you are able to alleviate the side effects with drugs, keep track of what works to use later. Somewhere along the way, some doctor may ask you if your child has had a specific chemotherapy drug. You will probably not remember all of them (or even be able to pronounce many of them), so having a list is helpful. You can make the list as detailed as fits your comfort level. You may also want to keep a three ring binder with lab results and test or scan reports. Being organized might not be the highest priority during treatment but it can reduce the stress level a bit to just have it all on hand in a binder.

As I read back in our journal, there are a few things that come to light over and over again that we had to deal with. Nausea was a big one. It took a couple rounds for us to figure out the best nausea medicine scheme for Nathan. We also noticed that the nausea got worse and lasted longer in each successive treatment. There was a cumulative effect. There are a few different drugs that work at varying levels depending on your child. We planned on Nathan getting some form of nausea medicine every six hours, and at five hours we were checking our watches to see how long we had until his next dose.

There is a cycle to chemotherapy and its corresponding side effects. It starts with administration of the chemotherapy cocktail. After a couple days your child starts to feel really bad. A couple more days and mouth sores may appear. At the same time, the blood counts drop. Sometimes red blood cells and platelets transfusions are needed. A few more days and things start to recover. Sores go away, blood counts rise, and your child starts to feel better. A week or so more of strengthening and your child repeats this cycle. The further into treatment you go, the longer this strengthening period may be.

As part of the chemotherapy cycle, the doctors kept a close eye on the blood counts or blood levels. Specifically the doctors are looking at hemoglobin, platelets, and absolute neutrophil count (ANC). Hemoglobin levels tell how many red blood cells are in the system. Low hemoglobin makes your child very tired and pale. Platelets are the part of the blood system that allows the blood to clot. If the platelets are low, it is hard for any cut or bruise to heal. Low platelets increase the risk of significant bleeding. Neutrophils are the white blood cells that are most critical to fighting germs. The ANC is a ratio of neutrophils to other white blood cells in the system. This ratio gives the doctors an idea of when your child is recovering from chemotherapy.

A child in chemotherapy is very susceptible to germs and viruses and are not equipped to fight them off. Therefore, it is important to keep your child away from germs you can avoid. We started calling ourselves "germ phobic" and would wash our hands constantly, have friends wash their hands before coming in the house, and anyone who was even remotely sick was not allowed near any of us. Friends understand. People who do not understand and do not help you are not necessary to have around your child. Nathan was very susceptible to host any bug that felt like visiting. He had many bouts of pneumonia, the flu, a staph infection, chicken pox, and respiratory infections. Each of these meant more time in the hospital to recover.

Even with these precautions, many times your child may still get sick from germs that they already have inside of them. You cannot always prevent your child from getting sick, but you can help. It is important to keep germs away, but it is more important to know how to handle things when your child does get sick, because they may. Find your hospital's procedures for your sick child and follow those. Here are some of ours:

- If your child gets sick during normal business hours, call the Oncology clinic not the Emergency Department (ED). The Oncology clinic is better suited to handle your issues and there are fewer germs there. Let the staff know if you are arriving sick, they may want to place you in an isolation room.
- For after business hours, know the phone number to the oncology doctor "on call"; write it in the front cover of your journal.
- Know the procedures for the ED and do not be afraid to use them. When oncology patients go to the ED they are allowed to bypass the waiting room and go straight to a patient room. Learn your hospitals procedures for a visit to the ED. The absolute best place to pick up unwanted germs is the hospital and mostly in the ED, not just the waiting room. Have your child wear a mask whenever not in their room to keep the germs out.
- Always have a bag packed and in the car for trips to the hospital. Each trip to the ED might result in an overnight stay at the hospital and many times a couple day stay. Every so often check the clothes and make sure they still fit and are seasonally appropriate. Have the bag include your toiletries and your child's. Have a favorite blanket and a loved stuffed animal. It is also good to include some new toy or activity they have not seen before and a book for you and quarters for the vending machines.
- Have a check list at the house of those things you have to pack last minute so you do not forget them. For example, the journal, video games, the favorite stuffed animal, laptop computer,

charging cables, and so on. Keep it on the refrigerator with a second copy in the journal.

- Do not hesitate to get your child to the hospital whenever things are not going correctly or when they need extra attention. If you catch things early enough, some problems can be handled at the clinic or with home care and you can avoid an exhausting trip to the hospital late at night. For example: it is very easy for the kids to get dehydrated. Many times we would take Nathan into the clinic because he was "droopy". The doctors would "juice him up" with fluids and the recovery was amazing.

ANC and Other Blood Counts

As mentioned before, one of the serious side effects of chemotherapy is reduction in the blood levels or "counts". When counts drop, specifically white blood cells (neutrophils), red blood cells (hemoglobin), and platelets, your child is at different types of risk. Each of these blood cells has a very important role in your child's health. Figure 3 shows a copy of a generic lab report for Nathan with the key results highlighted. Table 1 explains a little about each of the key results. Keep a binder with the lab results. It is helpful to keep track of labs when going through chemotherapy. As I mentioned, it tends to be a fairly predictable cycle. The sections below go into greater detail about the most important of these labs.

White blood cells, specifically neutrophils, are the body's army for fighting off germs and infections. These cells are the biggest defense your body has in its immune system. When neutrophils are low, or zero, (a condition called neutropenic) your child is at a greater risk of infections when they get them, there is little defense on their side to protect themselves. During and after each round of chemotherapy, the doctors take blood samples frequently to track the neutrophils and absolute neutrophil count (ANC). The ANC is calculated based on the total number of neutrophils with respect to the total number of white blood cells. It is very important to follow procedures exactly when your child's ANC is low. Confirm with your doctor what precautions they recommend and when you should go back to the hospital. Very little is more terrifying than your child having a 104 F fever with no white blood cells. Every moment of every day when Nathan was in this situation, I found myself praying that his counts would come back up before the fever got worse. The hospital staff was a constant support every time we ended up there, doing anything they could to help us through each battle.

The hemoglobin (HGB) in the blood carries oxygen throughout the body. When the HGB level drops, your child can get tired and act "scary sick". It becomes very easy for your child to develop a fever and become susceptible to other germs. When the HGB drops below a specific level identified by your oncology team, a transfusion of packed red blood cells is needed. The transfusion may take place in the clinic, the ED in some hospitals, or their hospital room. It can take as long as four hours to get the transfusion. Each hospital and medical staff have different procedures and guidelines. It generally takes about two hours per unit of cells. Early on your child will be tested for their blood type. It will be checked by the staff before the transfusion is given to your child. When Nathan was in active chemotherapy treatment he would have blood transfusions a few times for each round of therapy.

Platelets help blood clot. Low platelet levels make it easy to bleed and clotting is difficult. When the platelet levels drop too low, your child can get little spots all over their body called petechia. Petechia is a visual sign for you that your child might need a transfusion of platelets. As with the HGB level, your oncology team identifies a platelet level at which your child needs to have a platelet transfusion. Nathan had an adverse reaction the first time he received a platelet transfusion; he spiked a fever and broke out in hives. Subsequently, he was pre-medicated with acetaminophen (Tylenol) and diphenhydramine (Benadryl) prior to each platelet transfusion to prevent this reaction. The lab in the hospital may also "wash" the platelets for children with a more severe reaction. Keep note of these reactions somewhere prominent in your journal, perhaps with the list of medicines.

```
COMPREHENSIVE METABOLIC PROFILE
  SODIUM                  L 134       [138-145] mmol/L
  POTASSIUM               L 3.6       [3.7-5.6] mmol/L
  CHLORIDE                  98        [96-105]  mmol/L
  CARBON DIOXIDE, TOTAL
                           26.8       [20-28]   mmol/L
  GLUCOSE, RANDOM           95        [60-100]  mg/dL
  BLOOD UREA NITROGEN     H 24        [10-18]   mg/dL
  CREATININE                0.8       [0.4-1.1] mg/dL
  CALCIUM                 L 8.9       [9.0-11.0] mg/dL
  ALBUMIN                   4.1       [3.5-5.0] g/dL
  ALKALINE PHOSPHATASE      270       [101-335] U/L
  TOTAL BILIRUBIN         L 0.1       [0.2-1.0] mg/dL
  AST                       34        [0-45]    U/L
  TOTAL PROTEIN             6.8       [5.5-7.5] g/dL
  ALT                       50        [0-65]    U/L


DIRECT BILIRUBIN            <0.1      [0.0-0.4] mg/dL


MAGNESIUM                   2.0       [1.8-3.0] mg/dL


PHOSPHOROUS                 4.8       [3.6-6.5] mg/dL


CBC, HEMOGRAM
  WBC COUNT                 8.3       [4.0-12.0] x 10x3/mm3
  RBC COUNT               L 3.92      [4.00-5.30] x 10x6/mm3
  HEMOGLOBIN               12.4       [11.5-14.5] g/dL
  HEMATOCRIT               35.0       [32-42]   %
  MCV                      89.4       [76-90]   FL
  MCH                    H 31.6       [25-31]   pg
  MCHC                     35.3       [32-36]   g/dL
  RDW                      11.5       [11.5-14.5] %
  MPV                       7.2       [6.3-10.8] fL
  PLATELET COUNT            244       [140-440] x 10x3/mm3


CBC, DIFFERENTIAL
  SEGMENTED NEUTROPHIL      49        [32-54]   %
  LYMPHOCYTE               40.0       [27-57]   %
  MONOCYTE                  5.0       [0-5]     %
  EOSINOPHIL             H 6.0        [0-3]     %
  ABSOLUTE NEUTR. CNT.     4.07                 x 10x3/mm3
  RBC MORPHOLOGY         NORMOCHROMIC/NORMOCYTIC
```

Figure 3 Sample Lab Report

Table 1 Blood Counts Terminology

Blood Count	Explanation
WBC Count	White blood count. Includes all types of white cells and indicates potential to fight infections
Hemoglobin	Low hemoglobin indicates anemia
Platelet Count	Indicates the bloods ability to stop bleeding (or clot)
Absolute Neutrophil Count	Indicates number of white cells with the potential to fight bacterial infections
Serum Creatinine	Indicates renal function
Total Bilirubin	Indicates liver health
AST	Aspartate transaminase, indicates liver health
ALT	Alanine amino transferase, indicates liver health

Keeping Track of Medicines

While your child is in the hospital the staff there keeps track of all the medicines: when they were last given, when they are needed next, and the doses of all of them. When at home, you, the parents, need to do this. Some medicines are given twice a day, some three times, some every 6 hours, some every 8 hours, some just once, some at breakfast and others at dinner and still others "as needed". In some situations like ours now, we have different medicines depending on the timeline of his treatment. The first week has a timeline, the second week has a different timeline, and the third is still different. Add to this the complication of more than one person giving the medicines to the child and the task can be very daunting. We found the best way to keep and use all this information was with a spreadsheet. The spreadsheet has the times the medicines are due and doses, it can easily be checked off when given. If the medicine is already marked off, we know someone has given Nathan his medicines as indicated. We have our spreadsheet dated to remove even more ambiguity.

	Dosage	Sunday date	Monday date	Tuesday date	Wednesda date	Thursday date	Friday date	Saturday date
Medicine 1	5 ml	AM PM	AM PM	AM PM	AM PM	AM PM	AM PM	AM PM
Medicine 2	100 mg	AM	AM	AM	AM	AM	AM	AM
Medicine 3	5 mg	0800, 1600, 2400	0800, 1600, 2400	0800, 1600, 2400	0800, 1600, 2400	0800, 1600, 2400	0800, 1600, 2400	0800, 1600, 2400
Medicine 4	1 sqrt each nostril	AM	AM	AM	AM	AM	AM	AM
Medicine 5	400 mg	PM	PM	PM	PM	PM	PM	PM
Medicine 6	62.5mcg 1/2 tab	PM	PM	PM	PM	PM	PM	PM
Medicine 7	1/2 capful	bedtime	bedtime	bedtime	bedtime	bedtime	bedtime	bedtime

Figure 4 Medicine Schedule

Figure 4 shows an example of our medicine schedule. This spreadsheet is printed out every 3 weeks with the medicines for that time period. We tack them to the cupboard that contains all of Nathan's medicine so it is easy to mark. When we travel all the medicines and this schedule go into a single bag or box together. The doses are listed next to the medicine line giving a good reminder of exactly how much of each medicine is needed.

Hair Loss

Journal entry – *"Last night Nathan's hair started falling out. It is all over his pillow and me. I was kind of being quiet about it because I did not know if it would bother him. Well, when someone stopped by today they asked him about what was on his pillow. He said, "That's just my hair. It is falling out". I guess he knows and is not bothered by it."*

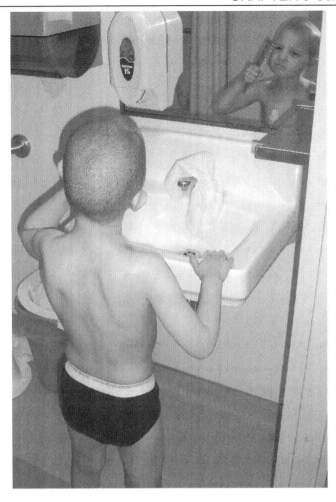

Hair loss is an ever present reminder of cancer. Many chemotherapy drugs can cause hair to fall out about a week after finishing the drug. We were uncertain how Nathan was going to handle his hair loss, especially the first time. Before his first round of chemotherapy, we had a hair cutting party at our house. Scott had his hair cut VERY short, Nathan had his hair cut, the boy next door had his hair cut, and Nathan's uncle and cousins cut their hair short so that Nathan would have other bald people around. When his short hair fell out on his pillow, Nathan was very nonchalant about it and had no issues being bald. It is my understanding that hair loss can be more traumatic for teenagers or girls. As parents it is best if you can down play the hair loss and help them with whatever form of head covering they want. Over the many years of treatment, Nathan's hair has come and gone frequently. There is little to do about it but make the child comfortable. Many children wear hats, scarves, etc. I'm sure older kids would wear wigs. Nathan just ignored it or just let it be. We had him in hats when out in the sun and would frequently just rub sunscreen on his bald head. I'm sure every child will probably be different with their hair.

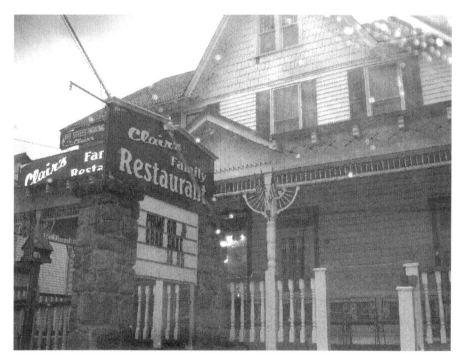

Figure 5 Claire's Family Restaurant

A bald head is considered a universal symbol for being on chemotherapy. People you meet along your journey deal with it in different ways. When traveling to the hospital for Nathan's MIBG therapy, we stopped in Morgantown, Pennsylvania, for dinner. We picked Claire's Family Restaurant. As we were eating our desert of strawberry pie, cherry crumb, or chocolate ice cream, the owner, a kind elderly man, stopped by to say hello. His name was Pop. He asked Nathan where his hair was. Then he looked at me and gently asked if it was just a haircut. I shook my head no. This man almost came to tears. Nathan was kindly answering his question; he was explaining to him that *"all that medicine those doctors keep giving me makes my hair fall out. And may I please have some chocolate sauce for my ice cream?"* Pop quickly returned with a whole lot of chocolate sauce and stayed to chat with us for a little bit. When we left to pay our bill Pop met us at the cash register and said that he wanted to *"take care of that"* for us. We resisted just a bit but then thanked him and continued on our way. Nathan was laughing and giggling the whole time. What a kind, sweet thing to do for strangers you will never see again.

Mouth Sores

Mouth sores can be a persistent and painful nuisance during chemotherapy treatments. A few days after starting a course of chemotherapy, your child may develop mouth sores. Mouth sores, or mucositis, are like canker sores throughout the mouth and down the throat and esophagus and through the entire intestinal tract to their bottom. They are extremely painful and pain medicines only dampen the pain, not remove it. The hospital staff gave us a recipe for mouthwash (recipe below) to help prevent or postpone the mouth sores. It only worked if we started it early enough and stayed with it. Different medical teams might have different medication they offer to help with mouth sores and sometimes you might need to try several of them to find what works for your child. Nathan preferred the home version and would therefore use it, which was the most important part. Remember the mouthwash works best as a preventative step; if the mouth sores showed up at all, it would be a tough week. It is very important to continue using the mouthwash even if mouth sores appear. It can help prevent a bacterial or fungal overgrowth in the mouth. This will help reduce the risk of an infection getting into the blood stream from the mouth sores. Work with your medical team to find the mouthwash solution that works for your child. It may be the home version, it may be the prescribed version, or it may be both. Use it after every meal and use it frequently BEFORE they start having mouth pain.

Once the sores started, there was no stopping them until Nathan's ANC started to climb. As soon as his neutrophil level recovered, they would help to heal the mouth sores. On many occasions the doctors would see Nathan's mouth sores shrinking and predicted that Nathan's ANC was coming back up even though the blood tests did not show it yet.

Mouthwash recipe

- Boil 2 quarts water
- Add 1 teaspoon salt
- Add 1 tablespoon baking soda
- Bring to boil
- Remove from heat
- Let cool
- Swish and spit after every meal
- Store in refrigerator
- Replace solution every week

Fevers

Fevers are a dangerous reality while your child is on chemotherapy. Fevers can identify bacterial infections or many other serious conditions. When your child's ANC is low (neutropenic) without the ability to fight the infection, and they have a fever, it is critical that your child is cared for by doctors at the hospital. Your medical team will have its definition of a fever for you and what you are to do when your child has one. Make sure you know the procedures and guidelines for when your child crosses this threshold. Make sure you know who to call, which can change depending on the time of day. Make sure you know what to do when you arrive at the ED. Many hospitals have a separate entrance for oncology patients.

For example, when Nathan spiked a fever we had our checklist to follow. (You will have your own procedure).

- Call the oncologist on call as soon as the fever went over 101 F (38.3 C) (or 100.4 F (38 C), depending on the hospital)
- Arrive at the Emergency Department (ED) within one hour of calling oncologist

- The ED staff take cultures from the central line and administer IV antibiotics within one hour of arriving at the hospital
- The ED staff will usually stay in contact with the oncologist on call and get instructions from them.
- Stay at the hospital until the fever is gone and the medical staff is comfortable with your child going home.

Here is a place to write some of your specifics:

Fever is defined as _____F (_____C)

Oncologist On Call Number: _____

Oncology Clinic Number: _____

These procedures are very important and potentially lifesaving. Many times, the fever will be just a fever with nothing life threatening and resolve in a few days. However, it always has the potential to be something a lot more serious. On at least two occasions, Nathan had pneumonia in one or both lungs. On another occasion, he had a bacterial infection in his central line. These infections can be critical to your child if left untreated while they are in the weakened condition that comes from cancer treatments.

Know your own medical team's protocol and follow it. The medical team in each of the hospitals in which Nathan was a patient had a slightly different set of instructions. Know them and write them in your journal. Have the "Oncologist On Call" phone number written in the front so you do not need to search for it when you need it. We always had one bag packed in the van so that once he spiked the fever, we only had to worry about getting him to the hospital and not whether we had clothes to wear, his special blankets he could not sleep at the hospital without, booties or slippers for Nathan, toys, and a stuffed animal to snuggle with.

Pain

Pain is a constant companion for cancer patients. Pain can come from many sources. There can be pain from disease in the bones making the bones ache. There can be pain when the treatment works because dying cancer cells become inflamed and swell in the bones. There can be pain because one spot in the body is so littered with disease that the joint is no longer round in its socket. There can be pain because cancer treatment hurts. Mouth sores hurt, nausea hurts, and it can just hurt all over, all the time. Pain is not to be ignored and your child should not be told to just tough it out. One cannot imagine all the pain that a child with cancer has to endure.

Many hospitals have a pain management team or a pain management plan for cancer patients. Use them. Even if your child is not a complainer, tough even when they do not need to be, don't ignore the fact they are still in pain. This means that you, as the parent, need to keep an eye on the pain level and look at other indicators as to how they are feeling. Make it your responsibility to ensure the other care givers know these signs; make sure they see them and take care of your child and the pain. Make sure that your pain management team deals with your child's specific type of pain, whether it is nerve pain, bone pain, etc.

We found out that there is a limit to the amount of pain medicine your child can take over a long period of time. During the weeks at the hospital prior to diagnosis Nathan was on a pain pump where he got a constant supply of medicine so he could simply function. After weeks of this he started having muscle tremors. Whenever he would relax enough to sleep his muscles would spasm and he could not fall asleep. All I could do was lie in bed with him and hold him to help him sleep. We spent many days and night like this with him completely wrapped in my arms while I cooed in his ear and rubbed the pain out of his arms, legs, back, anywhere I could reach.

Every child is different. Nathan had a lot of pain during treatment. When Nathan had a new regime of chemotherapy, he would have SEVERE leg pain. This usually led us to run additional scans to see if the disease was progressing and growing. For Nathan these intense pain bouts were followed by a significant (by my standards) reduction in disease. In every case, it was difficult to try and determine what was causing the pain. The best thing we could do was to try to manage the pain with whatever methods were available to us. There are many pain medicines available, and they can be administered in different ways. Work with the pain management teams to find the best one for your child. Do not have your child work through the pain. There is no need for it; there are medicines to help.

Journal entry - *"Today Nathan continued to whine about his throat hurting. This is reasonable considering the mouth sores. I told him he had some Miracle mouthwash that would make his throat go numb and would not hurt for a bit. He refused, of course, he hated taking medicine. So I told him if he whined about his throat hurting again he was swishing this medicine around his mouth. So, suddenly his throat did not hurt, but both his legs ached. I could rub them; there is no medicine for that. When questioned about all this, he admitted his throat was the problem, but he did not have to take yucky medicine for achy legs. "*

Remember to be a kid

One of the easiest and hardest things to do during our journey was to remember that Nathan was just a kid. He was only 3 ½ years old when diagnosed. Here are some of my favorite journal entries.

Journal entry - *"Today I think is classified as a good day. Kate and I arrived at the hospital to see Nathan running down the hall after a silly putty ball that he had thrown. The funniest part was Grandpa running after him trying to keep up with the medicine tower (what we affectionately call R2D2). I think we have his pain management under control finally. He had a good few hours before he got tired. This included swinging on the outside swing. Great smiles."*

Journal entry – *"I picked Nathan up at school and we walked down the hall to see Miss Judy (he wanted a sucker and some snuggling). When she was not there we argued about which way to go. I wanted to go the long way inside while he wanted to go the long way outside. It was snowing. So, I started walking to the door singing "I'm the line leader". This brought the appropriate response of my child sprinting past me saying "No you're not". Then he touched the door, laid his head back* and gave an appropriate maniacal laugh. "Ha, ha, ha". Do your best ghoulish laugh. I died laughing and am still now as I repeat this."

Journal entry – "Today we re-instituted Tether Dinosaur, the famous game where you tie a plastic dinosaur to the string of the blinds and whack it with a bigger plastic dinosaur…hours of fun for your soon-to-be four-year-old. Nathan also continued to perfect his skill with twenty-something nurses. Today it was Kelly who got the moves put on her. At one point, I heard that he was on her lap being fed grapes and watching his favorite show…whatever that happens to be today. That's my boy!"

Journal entry – "About one minute after returning home from dropping Nathan off at school, I get a call from Nathan's school director. Nathan was in her office crying that his legs hurt. Back into the car with my trusty pain medicine and off to school. When I arrived Nathan and the director were having a lot of fun reading stories in the office. No pain to be found. I gave the meds and explained that the reason I was hoping Nathan could attend all day today was because this is probably his last day until February or March. Nathan then interjected that he did not want to stay "all day" just lunch, nap and the afternoon."

Journal entry – "Nathan has told me all that the tooth fairy is supposed to accomplish tonight. She is to come to his room and find the tooth under his pillow. Then she will take it to her palace where she will do something with it and we do not know what it is. He says she will leave a piece of money (a quarter) under his pillow. He thinks that since this is his first lost tooth that she might also leave him a stuffed cat; hint, hint tooth fairy. This is all he wants to say to the tooth fairy. "Please take my tooth and take good care of it and write me back to tell me what you did with it." – Nathan"

Stem Cell Harvest

Stem cells are small immature cells that can become any type of blood cell. During some treatments such as bone marrow transplant, the bone marrow can be damaged such that it needs to be rescued by these stem cells. Stems cells may be collected several ways. One of them is through the blood stream after receiving stem cell mobilizing medication. Stem cells captured from the blood are called peripheral blood hematopoietic stem cells (or peripheral stem cells for short).

On our protocol, after two rounds of chemotherapy, peripheral stem cells were harvested to be stored for future use after high dose chemotherapy. Stem cells can remain frozen for many years and can be used when they are needed. At this point in the treatment time line, the disease had been reduced enough that the danger of capturing cancer cells during a stem cell harvest procedure is very low. To collect the cells, a larger catheter was surgically implanted in the large neck vessel to harvest the stem cells from the blood stream. A very large machine was attached to the catheter and over a few hours the machine collected stem cells and returned other blood cells back in to the blood stream. Stem cell harvesting can take up to five days to get the number of stem cells recommended. After completion the catheter was removed. The stem cells were checked for infection and tumor presence and stored for use later. Nathan did pretty well with this procedure. It only took two sessions to successfully harvest plenty of stem cells that were used months later during his bone marrow transplants.

Scans

During this long winding road of childhood cancer treatment, there are plenty of scans and tests performed. Most scans tell the current state of the disease. They also can tell how your child is recovering from treatment and how their body is reacting to it. The following sections give a brief overview of each scan or test that Nathan had. Each section tells what the scan identifies, how it is performed, and insights we learned through Nathan's experience. In general they are in the order in which he first received them.

The most important bit of advice I can give applies to all scans and tests. In every case make sure you know what you, as a parent, need to do to make the scan or test as accurate as possible. Talk to the doctors or technicians to make sure you and your child are prepared for each scan.

Managing Scan Information

There are many scans and lab tests and their reports to keep organized. As mentioned before a three ring binder works well. It is always a good idea to understand what the scans and tests say. Most of the information may or may not make complete sense to you, but, over time, some of the words become familiar and you start to notice those terms that mean the most. It is useful when you have to work with multiple hospitals and doctors to know what scans and tests have been performed and where. It may prevent your child from having a scan or test repeated unnecessarily.

One thing we learned a few months into Nathan's journey is to always get your own copy of the scans and reports. The hospital must give you a copy when you ask for one. This is true for electronic as well as written test results. Keep the electronic disks together and place the written reports in a binder where they can be easily found and used. More than once, having an electronic copy in our possession helped speed up the resolution of issues. We have worked with five hospitals. We have been able to bring copies of the scans and reports with us to the new hospital. Since we brought them, the new hospital did not need to request them from the old hospital. Therefore there was no delay in evaluation and treatment.

Having your own copy of the scan reports can also help you remember what you saw or were told by the doctors. It gives you time to review information and allow you to ask educated questions the next time you see the doctors. We had another way to remember what the scans showed. When in the room observing the scan, you can sometimes see the image on the screen while it is running. You are not allowed to ask the technicians any questions that relate to your child's scan or diagnosis, but, you can, from memory, draw what you saw. I always had the journal with me and drew what I saw as best I could, and I am no artist. These sketches have come in handy. On at least two occasions, while waiting for scan results that were taking longer than expected, the doctor told me that they were looking at a "new spot". I reviewed my own notes and was able to tell when I had seen that spot before. It gave the doctors and technicians the scan date to confirm it was not new. In both of these instances, it happened when we went to a new hospital and the staff was not yet completely familiar with Nathan's scan history.

CT Scan

A computed tomography or CT scan is a detailed scan. CT scans are used for many medical situations, not just neuroblastoma evaluation. CT scans use slices of x-rays put together to create a 3D image of your child. This scan allows the doctors to see in detail an area that may have disease or some other concern. CT scans are usually done in sections of the body and not an entire body image unless necessary. Make sure you know what preparation is needed for the CT scan. Sometimes the child needs to not eat before it (this is called NPO). Most times there is a contrast dye injection, and the child needs to be "accessed" or have a way to inject the dye either in their port or through a peripheral IV in their arm.

Nathan's first CT scan was done at the local children's hospital. Prior to diagnosis, the doctors were having his abdomen and pelvis scanned to determine why he was having hip pain. The scan stopped an inch or two from the top of his kidneys. Unfortunately for us, Nathan's tumor was on top of his left kidney. However, this only delayed diagnosis by a week or so.

MRI

Magnetic Resonance Imaging (MRI) is also a detailed scan. It is also used for many medical situations. It uses a large magnet to image the soft tissues of the body. There is usually an injection of a "contrast" dye to help make the images brighter. An MRI does not use radiation to acquire the images.

Nathan usually had an MRI to investigate an "area of interest" on an MIBG scan. The advantage of the MRI is that it does not use radiation, and after so many scans we are trying to minimize his radiation exposure.

Bone Scan

A bone scan is a nuclear medicine scan designed to show the places in a person's bones that are growing rapidly or have high levels of activity, such as a healing broken bone or growth plates. It is not a scan specific to your child's cancer or any cancer. The technicians inject a radioactive dye that is absorbed by the bones, the more dye that is absorbed in a specific area the more activity there is in that area. The areas of increased activity will be highlighted in the image; in the images shown in this book, they are the darkened areas. However, scans can just as easily be viewed with the high activity areas being light on a dark background. If the scan is normal the growth plates at the ends of each bone are the darkest, as shown in Figure 6. When the scan is not normal, there can be high activity levels in other areas where there is boney disease as seen in Figure 7. In this figure, you can see darkened areas in his skull. There is also extra activity in his right hip and his ribs. Again, it takes practice and experience to determine exactly where the scans are abnormal; we rely on the radiologist for that.

The bone scan is most useful when the disease is highly active in the bones, as it would be during diagnosis if your child has disease in their bones. If your child has only soft tissue disease, the bone scan will look perfectly normal. In Figure 7 you can see darkened areas in the skull, ribs, and throughout the skeleton. Very quickly, in less than a year, these areas appeared normal on the bone scan as can be seen in the Figure 6. However, his disease was still there five years later and was clearly seen on the MIBG scan.

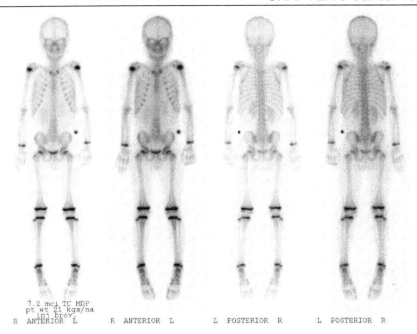

Figure 6 Nathan's "Normal" Bone Scan

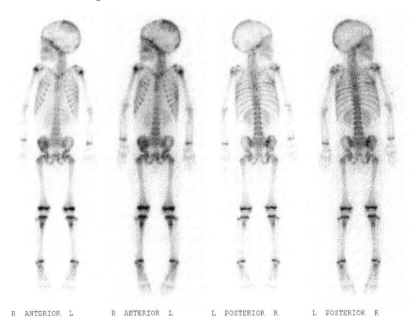

Figure 7 Nathan's Original Bone Scan

Metaiodobenzylguanidine (MIBG) Scan

The MIBG scan is a nuclear medicine scan specific to neuroblastoma. The patient is injected with Metaiodobenzylguanidine. The I in MIBG is radioactive Iodine. Once injected, the neuroblastoma absorb the MIBG dye. It was described to me that "they eat it like candy". After 24 hours the patient is placed on a scanner and the radiation levels are recorded. The darkened areas on the scan (Figure 8) are the locations of the MIBG dye. The dark areas can be neuroblastoma or places that normally "uptake" the MIBG dye. There is one caution to the MIBG scan: some neuroblastoma may be MIBG negative and do not absorb the dye. That does not mean there are no neuroblastoma cells there; it just means you cannot see them with this scan.

There are usually three types of scans performed during a session. The first is a full body view. There are sensors above and below the child. As the scan is performed, the table the child is on slides into the scanner and a two dimensional view is created, as shown in Figure 8. After a short break, the three dimensional scan is performed. The child stays in the same position as the scanner rotates around them. The scanner takes slices all the way around the child. The computer creates a three dimensional scan that the radiologist can rotate on the computer to get a better image of area of interest and determine if it is normal uptake of MIBG or disease. It is also common to take lateral skull images if there is disease in the head, shown in Figure 10. An image of Nathan on an MIBG scanner can be seen in Figure 11.

As mentioned, the dark areas on the scan are the locations of the MIBG dye. There are some normal places the MIBG is absorbed, the liver, the heart, some glands, and urine for instance. Anything on the image that looks like a bone is neuroblastoma in the bones, also called boney disease. Figure 8 shows a relatively clean 2-D MIBG scan. It is easy to pick out the port as the dark spot in the chest. The glands in the head/face are normal and show in each scan. The large dark area in the abdomen shaped like a weird triangle is the liver. Below that is the bowels. These areas are usually fuzzy. And finally if you look really close you can see disease in his femurs, tibias and right hip, identified with NB in the figure.

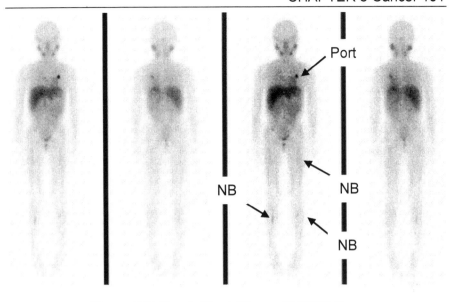

Figure 8 Nathan's Most "Normal" MIBG Scan

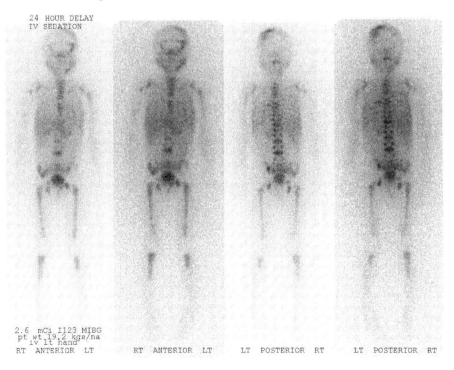

Figure 9 Figure 10 Nathan's Original MIBG Scan

Figure 9 and Figure 10 show Nathan's first MIBG scans. You can see a lot of activity throughout his skeleton. There are "hot spots" in his skull, ribs, shoulders, legs, arms and spine. His hands and feet seem to be clear. When you compare this scan to the bone scan, Figure 7, you can see the activity correlates between the two of them. As I mentioned, within a year the bone scan looked normal, but this MIBG scan still showed wide spread disease. The lateral skull images, Figure 10, shows activity behind the eyes and on top of the skull. There were very few places the MIBG scan did not show disease. We were told the reason the primary tumor and the liver were not glowing very much in Figure 9 was because the rest of the disease had "eaten" all the MIBG dye before it could be absorbed.

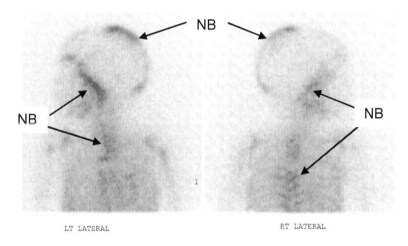

Figure 10 Nathan's Original MIBG Scan - Lateral Skull Images

MIBG scans can be performed at most hospitals that treat neuroblastoma. Each hospital may have a slightly different MIBG scanner and therefore a slightly different final image. Figure 11 shows Nathan in an MIBG scanner. MIBG is not an exact scan. The images can be fuzzy because of the "free" iodine not absorbed in the system. There is no "anatomy" in the MIBG image to refer to so it is difficult to decide exactly where each spot located and if it is supposed to be there. The radiologists that read these scans have read enough of them that their experience is what you rely on for guidance and insight.

If the radiologist identifies an area as disease and more information is needed, additional scans might be performed (such as an MRI) to confirm whether the spot is disease or just a shadow. Some scanners have a CT scanner built in the same machine as does the machine shown in Figure 11. In this machine, after the hour long MIBG scan Nathan will stay very still and the machine performs a small dose CT image over it giving anatomy to the blurry images helping the radiologists obtain a more accurate reading.

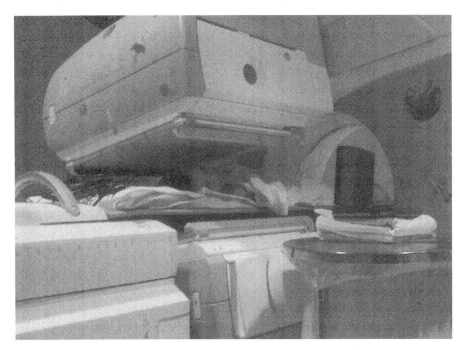

Figure 11 Nathan in MIBG Scanner with CT Imaging

Glomerular Filtration Rate (GFR)

The glomerular filtration rate, or nuclear GFR, tells the doctors your child's renal function. It gives an indication of how long it takes the kidneys to flush chemicals or medicines out of your child's body. The lower the GFR, the slower the kidneys are working and the longer the drugs remain in the body.

The GFR is performed by injecting a known quantity of a radioactive material into your child. After a given time, a blood sample is taken to see how much of the chemical has been removed. A second sample is taken some time later. From these samples it is determine the rate in which the material is removed. Many treatment protocols have a GFR limit for the amount of treatment drugs that can be given. If the GFR is below a specific level, your child may be given a smaller dose of medication because the drug will be in their system longer and therefore be impacting your child longer. If the GFR is too low and your child is given the same dose as a normal GFR, then you can potentially be overdosing the child on chemotherapy or other treatment, creating what is called toxicity.

There can be some ambiguity on how the GFR is performed. Hospitals do it differently and give different instructions on how much the child should eat or drink while waiting for the samples to be taken. Make sure you clarify with the technician running the test or the doctor overseeing the test exactly what is expected of you and your child. Find out if the child should be on IV fluids, see how much they should drink while waiting, ask whether they can eat, and whether they are allowed to run around. As with all tests and scans, Make sure you know what you, as a parent, need to do to insure the scan or test is as accurate as possible.

One time I remember being a bit too lax in my preparation for Nathan's GFR test just before his Bone Marrow Transplant. We had done GFR before and I really didn't pay any attention to how Nathan should prepare for the GFR sampling or even what the test results would be used for. I did not know if he should drink water, if he could run around, or any other activities that might affect the outcome. Nathan's GFR had always been high, so I did not worry about it. Then the test came back and his was very low. And worse, I didn't even know this mattered at the time. I was very quickly enlightened on the importance of the GFR test. Since the test was so low, we allowed Nathan's kidneys to rest a couple weeks and then retested his GFR. The next test was higher, but still showed Nathan's kidneys weakened. This test impacted Nathan's treatment level in MIBG therapy and bone marrow transplant. Nathan was given a reduced amount of therapy drug in both cases. This test let the doctors know that, at that point in time, his kidneys could NOT accept a full dose of either drug without putting him in jeopardy of severe toxicities because the drugs would be in his system longer than desired due to a reduction in kidney function. The biggest lesson I learned from this experience is that scans are always run with a purpose in mind. It is my job to make sure I know what the scan is for and how Nathan should act while getting the scan.

Bone Marrow Biopsy and Aspirations

Bone marrow biopsy and aspiration are performed to determine if there is disease in the bone marrow. It is an invasive procedure. And your child will be put under anesthesia. The doctors put a hollow needle in the pelvic bone and take out a core sample of bone marrow from the pelvic bone and also draw out some liquid bone marrow (it looks like blood). Once the child recovers from the anesthesia, they should stay calm so that they do not bleed too much. The biggest risk is infection at the site which can easily be avoided by keeping the bandages on and the site clean. Each child will have a different reaction to anesthesia. Many children are groggy all day, or have a headache or body aches, or they may just feel cruddy. Other kids are not affected for very long and want to run around like normal. It is important that they do not run around and are kept calm and sitting. The more activity they do, the bigger chance the bandages will get full and fall off, leading to a potential for infection.

I remember Nathan's first bone marrow biopsy; it was performed as part of his diagnosis, before we knew what we were dealing with. Nathan was scheduled for the procedure early in the day. Since he was going to be anesthetized he was not allowed to eat (this is called NPO). The surgery time came and went. Scott, Nathan, and I were in a tiny pre-operative room trying to distract Nathan as best we could. Hours later a nurse came in and asked us if we wanted to see clergy. I muttered, "*Sure,*" not really feeling comfortable about meeting clergy I did not know. I explained to Scott, who was in my snuggle spot on Nathan's bed, what the nurse had asked. He immediately asked if maybe she meant Dennis, our pastor. I walked into the hall to tell the nurse that yes; I would love to see *"our clergy,"* and down the hall came Dennis our pastor. What a relief. From that point on, we knew that no matter what was going on, our church family would be there to help even if we did not know we needed help and did not ask for any. They were a support we leaned on heavily for many years. Not surprising they didn't seem to mind the weight at all.

HVA and VMA

Homovanillic acid (HVA) and vanillylmandelic acid (VMA) are two acids found in your child's urine at small normal levels. Most neuroblastoma cells excrete these two acids into the blood stream. Therefore, you can often tell the status of disease activity by measuring the level of these two acids; the higher the levels, the higher the activity of the neuroblastoma. Unfortunately, some neuroblastoma is HVA and VMA negative. In those cases, this test will not be an accurate indication of disease status. The test is completed with a urine sample. Some hospitals have the urine collected over a 24 hour period; others do it with a random sample.

There are a couple draw backs to this test. First VMA can be falsely elevated in your child's system if they eat vanilla within a few days of the test. Because of this, vanilla should be avoided before this test. This may seem like a simple thing to do until you remember the vanilla ice cream available in most hospital freezers. There are other things that can elevate VMA but they are not as readily available as vanilla ice cream. Second, it can take one to two weeks to get the test results back from the lab. You should have other test results back well before you receive this one.

One more point of interest is that we found each lab that runs the HVA/VMA tests has different normal levels. Make sure you look at the child's results compared to the "normal" level from each lab. Nathan's doctors also mentioned that HVA/VMA can be a "lagging" indicator, meaning there would be other indicators before this one that his disease was progressing or improving. For us, as the HVA/VMA levels dropped over time, it was an obvious indicator showing Nathan's disease going away.

MIBG Therapy

As mentioned above, an MIBG scan is when the radioactive dye Metaiodobenzylguanidine (MIBG) is injected into the body. Neuroblastoma soak up this dye. The next day, the child is put under a scanner that measures where the dye is located, thus showing the doctors the location of the neuroblastoma. If your child's disease is MIBG positive, MIBG dye at higher doses can be used to treat your child. A more radioactive isotope of iodine is used for treatment compared to the one used for imaging. The MIBG treatment can have a significant impact on the disease load. However, it has been shown that it needs to be performed in conjunction with other therapies to completely remove the disease as part of frontline therapy. Due to the radioactive nature of the therapy, MIBG treatment requires very specific rooms and guidelines; therefore, there are only a few hospitals in the United States that perform MIBG therapy. Work with your doctors and insurance company to pick the right one for your family.

Sample MIBG Treatment Timing

MIBG treatment was surprisingly simple for us as a family. Many treatments are painful, intense, and long. MIBG therapy involved a lot of precautions and a lot of training, but the treatment was straight forward and short. The worst side effect of the intense MIBG therapy was that it would wipe out Nathan's bone marrow such that it would no longer be able to produce blood cells. However, so does conditioning chemotherapy for the bone marrow transplant (BMT) which was to follow MIBG therapy. In Nathan's protocol these two treatments were timed in a way that this effect would happen together.

The treatment timeline may differ depending on the therapy plan you are following. Each child's therapy can be personalized. Nathan's treatment timeline went like this:

- Monday: admitted to hospital
- Tuesday: A catheter is inserted in the bladder while Scott and I received training on caring for a radioactive child. The nurses

would not be entering the room unless absolutely necessary. The IV pole was placed right next to the room door so the nurses and staff can access it when needed.

- Tuesday afternoon: MIBG treatment injection
- Wednesday and Thursday: Nathan was radioactive and had minimal contact with anyone. Scott and I alternated as care givers, with only one of us in the room at a time. There were serious restrictions on parents and visitors, but Nathan could rest and play video games, watch TV, etc. Anything that could be done while staying in bed.
- Friday: released
- Saturday: drove home

When MIBG therapy is administered in conjunction with Bone Marrow Transplant (BMT), like we did, the next week is spent at home. This part was very surreal to us that Nathan had gone through this tough treatment that was going to wipe out his bone marrow and here he was at home just waiting to admit to the hospital for the BMT phase of treatment.

Nathan's immune system and numbers would no longer be improving. Over the next couple weeks the blood counts went to zero from MIBG therapy, right at about the same time his "conditioning" chemotherapy had him bottom out for his BMT. He would then receive his stem cells back and start the recovery process. BMT and recovery are discussed in detail in the BMT section.

MIBG Treatment Specifics

MIBG treatment is a radioactive therapy that needs to be given under radiation precautions and guidelines. The child stays in a lead lined room. The child's room is covered with paper and plastic. There are lead walls between the child's bed and the parent's sleeping area. Usually, the areas are separated with some distance to protect the parents from radiation exposure. With all this lead in the room, we were told that the radiation should not be able to get through plastic such as our gloves. If the guidelines for the parents are followed, their radiation exposure should be about the same as a normal x-ray. Direct contact with the child or any of their fluids can be dangerous to you.

Visitations to see the child are strictly limited. Only one person is allowed in the room at a time. If a visitor enters the room, the parent leaves. The simplest way to follow this is to not have visitors for this treatment. This is safer and easier for all. Check with your hospital for their rules and restrictions. Visitors may be welcome, just expect some precautionary procedures to be in place. In general this treatment was short and simple and out of town, which made it easier to not have any visitors during the time in the lead lined room.

Nathan slept through the entire process of the MIBG injection. Scott was not in the room during the injection since the technician was. Nathan's radiation levels were the highest over the first few hours. Scott was told to not touch him and stay behind the large lead shields. We were instructed initially to not bring anything that Nathan would want to take home because, after using it, the item would be radioactive and it would be thrown out. However, once there, we found out that if you put things in plastic bags he could keep them. Nathan was very peculiar with this rule. He brought to treatment the white teddy bear that was given to him by the MIBG manufacturer. Nathan had not really played with the bear before treatment; it didn't even have a name. We figured it was an appropriate use for the MIBG bear. Once there, this bear was now *"My favorite,"* and, *"I must take this home,"* kind of bear. A little extra plastic was placed on the bear and he got loved on and then was taken home.

While in the hospital for MIBG therapy, Nathan was placed on a sedative drip to reduce his activity level and allow him to stay in bed and calm for the days he was radioactive. Versed is an IV drug that has a calming effect and can cause a child to forget the treatment time. The Versed drip worked wonderfully for Nathan. He was able to spend hours lying on his bed playing with his video game. He could watch movies and nap. During most visits to the hospital, he is constantly running around the room when he feels well. It would have been very difficult to keep our four year old calm for two days without it. Again, check with your doctors to see if this is part of your MIBG treatment; it may not be standard in all hospitals, but we highly recommend it. Nathan only remembers the baseball game we attended the day before treatment began.

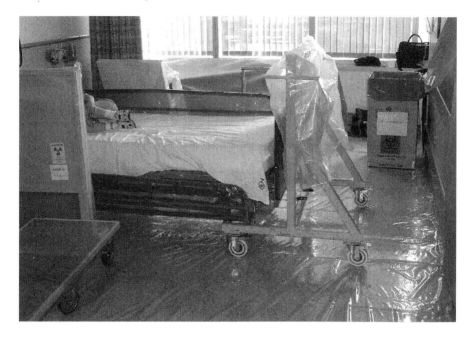

Figure 12 Nathan lying in bed in his MIBG Therapy room

Being Radioactive

When your child is released from the hospital they will still be radioactive, but will be below EPA standards. There are many things to be careful about: no kissing, no long term close exposure (such as sitting on your lap while watching a movie), and flushing twice after they go potty. Make sure to get all the precautions before leaving the hospital. Read them and follow them. Make sure you understand the potential risk of exposure to yourself and the side effects you may experience.

Journal entry - *After Nathan left the hospital we took a short trip to the park. Nathan had a complete blow out in his pants. Normally, this would not be too tough, but he was still radioactive. This just gave a new perspective on how different our life had become.*

Radiation Treatment

Neuroblastoma is considered to be a radiation sensitive form of cancer. This means neuroblastoma should be killed with radiation therapy. Therefore, radiation is another "big gun" in treating neuroblastoma. Radiation treatment follows recovery from bone marrow transplant. Radiation treatment is a targeted therapy, where you decide the locations to treat and it generally only affects those areas. In many neuroblastoma cases, it is clear where the treatment should be targeted, such as the primary tumor bed, the "hottest" metastatic area, or any other location that may have residual disease. Other times it is less clear, such as when there is too much disease to radiate it all, or there is still bulky disease remaining. In this case you, the oncologist and the radiation oncologist work together to decide how much disease should be radiated, if any.

Radiation treatment requires your child to lie perfectly still for a few minutes. Nathan's treatments were about ten minutes long, including setup time. You and your doctors decide if your child can take the radiation treatments while awake or whether they need to be anesthetized. Can they stay still that long, even if their head is bolted to the table? Each option has its pros and cons. Talk with your primary oncologist and radiation oncologist to make the right choice for your child. If your child is awake during treatment, there is a short recovery after each treatment. Additionally, without anesthesia, there is no need to keep your child from eating before treatment. However, many small children cannot lie still for the duration of the treatment. If radiation is targeted at the skull, a mask bolts the head to the table so the head cannot move. For little kids, having a face mask bolted to a table may just be too much. If this is the case, there is always the option to use anesthesia. In addition, depending on your circumstances, radiation therapy may be performed on an outpatient basis. Work with your team to make the best decision for your child.

After BMT, Nathan still had bulky disease remaining throughout his skeleton. Irradiating all of it was NOT an option. With the help of his oncologist and radiation oncologist, we chose to have radiation treatments on three different sections of disease: his right and left tibias and the skull. We were not sure if radiation was going to be effective enough to radiate more areas, so we chose the ones we felt would be the most useful with the least amount of harm to Nathan's skeleton. We specifically avoided irradiating his growth plates.

Nathan had radiation treatment twice a day for ten days. His treatment timeline was on five days, off two days, on five days. He was required to lie perfectly still on a metal table for about five minutes each round. In order to make sure his head stayed perfectly still a mask was made for his face and his head was bolted to the table. In Figure 13 note the face mask and stuffed cat. Most four year old children must be anesthetized for radiation therapy. We had a terrible time trying to work out all the arrangements for getting anesthesia. If Nathan could lie still for the treatment time he would not need the anesthesia. Having two treatments a day made anesthesia difficult at best, especially if we wanted Nathan to eat anything.

We were able to get the radiation doctor to agree to let Nathan try to a test case without anesthesia. Our first attempt at this failed miserably, but I think we were asking too much of Nathan. During the trial run, he had to lie there while they measured the position for treatment. He had to stay still while they ran a mock CT scan. He had to continue to remain still while they made the mask on his face and it hardened. And, finally, he was asked to lie still while they simulated treatment. It was just not possible. He was four. You must give the child an opportunity to succeed; in this case we did not. After failing a second time to get everyone we needed together for him for anesthesia, we tried another trial run to see if Nathan could succeed without anesthesia. This time we just simulated him staying still for treatment duration. This time he did fine.

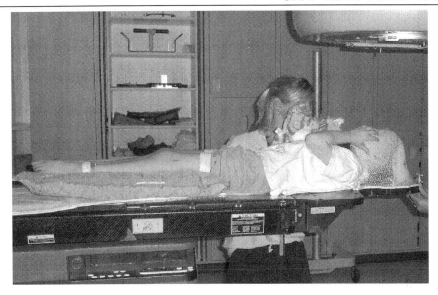

Figure 13 Nathan Ready for Radiation Therapy

Nathan was very bribable with stuffed cats or other toys. He had a difficult time with radiation at first. We had asked him to lie still on a table for ten minutes twice a day with his head bolted to a table while wearing a mask. After the second round, the technicians mentioned they had a toy cabinet and asked if Nathan would like something. He chose a stuffed cat. Before the following round, Nathan asked about the toy cabinet. They did have another stuffed cat, but it was the last one. This round he was a perfect angel, knowing that cat was there for him. That evening Scott visited the toy store and rounded up as many small stuffed cats as he could. They worked wonders. Nathan did the remaining radiation treatments doing exactly what was asked of him. Each time he received a new stuffed cat of his choice. When we were done with his very last radiation treatment, the technicians gave him a VERY large stuffed white tiger as a going away present. The stuffed tiger is still on his bed. He sleeps with it every night and remembers NONE of his radiation treatments.

Immunotherapy

Chemotherapy is a widespread therapy that treats the entire body to kill cancer cells. Immunotherapy (or biologic therapy) is a targeted therapy where it targets specific cells in the body. Immunotherapy finds a way to change the cancer cells so the body (immune system) will kill them. The reason your body does not fight cancer on its own is because it does not see the cancer as foreign and, therefore, does not do anything about it. If the body could see the cancer cells as foreign, then the body would help kill them. There are a few approaches to achieving this. One way is to convince the cancer cells themselves to stop being dangerous, by dying or maturing into normal cells. Another is to mark the cell as foreign and let the body attack it. Immunotherapy has been shown to work best on minimal disease, sometimes called "minimal residual disease," and generally does not work well on bulky disease. Therefore, this type of treatment is used after the harsher and more standard forms of chemotherapy. The next few sections describe the immunotherapy that Nathan had during his cancer treatments.

Acutane – Cis Retinoic Acid

Cis Retinoic Acid is a medicine designed to treat acne. I'm not sure who thought of using an acne medicine to fight cancer, but I'm sure glad they did. As I understand it, each cell in your body has working parts inside the cell and receptors on the outside of the cell. These receptors are places where other cells can connect to and tell it things. For example, there is a receptor that tells a cancer cell it is perfectly healthy and should reproduce as much as it can. There is another receptor where the Cis Retinoic Acid connects that tells the cancer cell it is no longer healthy and should stop dividing and making more cells. It does not kill the cell, but it stops it from being so dangerous

Cis Retinoic Acid is given in six courses at the end of frontline therapy. This treatment is pretty easy on the child, with minimum adverse side effects. It is a single pill taken daily. There is plenty of paper work and warnings to sign before treatment can begin. Cis Retinoic Acid has been shown to have severe side effects on a fetus if the patient is pregnant and taking it. Therefore ALL patients taking this drug must sign or have a parent sign the warning documents, even for a four year old boy. Generally, your child will only need additional monitoring of their kidney functions.

This drug was very tough on Nathan. The most obvious side effect was it made his skin REALLY dry. It was worse than I could have imagined dry skin ever being. Lotions and creams were a must and they only prevented the skin from cracking. The worse side effect was his mood. Cis Retinoic Acid made him moody to the point he could not control his emotions or reactions. He would be smiling one minute, angry the next, and crying shortly thereafter. Nathan's side effects got worse and worse with each course. His mood swings got less predictable, not more predictable. It was one of those times when we chose to just push through the treatment and not try to fix him or make the symptoms go away. We chose to lighten his load and let him go relax more and not really hound him for his bad behavior. Once the therapy was over he returned to his normal delightful self. We did learn from this. There are other drugs that can make him mean and moody, but we can now see the signs and realize it is not really him doing it but the effects of the medicine and treat him accordingly.

Antibodies

One of the receptors on the outside of a cancer cell is called the GD2 receptor. Antibodies treatments use the GD2 receptor to attack the cancer. It is assumed that most neuroblastoma cells are GD2 positive, which means the neuroblastoma cell has a GD2 receptor the antibody therapy can attach to. When the antibody cell attaches to the receptor, the body then sees the foreign antibody and attacks it. The immune system kills the antibody and the cancer cell it is attached too. In the best case scenario, the body learns not only to kill the antibody but to attack the cancer cell whether or not the antibody is still attached to it. In this way, the body can learn to kill cancer cells directly.

Antibody therapy has many side effects. It was one of the most difficult treatments that Nathan received. The antibodies attach to the GD2 receptor, which is found on most nerve cells. Therefore, when the antibodies are attaching to the cancer cells it is irritating ALL the nerve cells in the body. This is a different type of pain than any other he had during treatments; it was horrible. He was given pain medicines in high doses to control it. The pain medicines made him really mean. An interesting twist to antibody therapy is this pain is a good sign, not a bad one. If the child is in pain, then the antibodies are getting to their target. If the child does not have pain, the child's immune system has created its own antibody that kills the treatment before it can help. This puts a parent in a very tough emotional spot. First, you hate to see your child in pain. However, if he is not in pain then the treatment is not working at all. I did not enjoy antibody therapy at all, however, I feel sure it did help in the fight against cancer.

Nathan had a worse side effect than the pain. After several rounds of antibodies, Nathan developed an allergic reaction to the antibody treatment and got hives in his throat during the injection. His throat would start closing up, and he could not breathe. He was given oxygen and medication breathing treatments to help him breathe. We then remained in the hospital for a couple hours after treatment for his oxygen levels to stabilize.

Each day after antibody therapy, Nathan was a complete mess. He was tired and angry from the treatment and the pain medicine. Then he was jittery and agitated from the multiple breathing treatments. We would take him back to the Ronald McDonald house and see him just sit there watching the other kids do things. During most of the treatments, there were other kids on the same cycle that he was, and Nathan would sit with one of them, seeming perfectly content to have a friend and watch the world go by. All we could do was try to make him as happy as possible. This was usually accomplished with a visit from his cousin. It is amazing what her smile and a package of chicken nuggets could do for Nathan's well-being.

NOTES

Fever is defined as _____**F (**_____**C)**

Oncologist On Call Number: _____

Oncology Clinic Number: _____

_____

_____

_____

_____

_____

_____

_____

_____

_____

_____

_____

_____

_____

_____

_____

_____

_____

NOTES

CHAPTER 4. BONE MARROW TRANSPLANT

Bone marrow transplant (BMT), also called stem cell rescue, is the longest and most difficult part of the treatment timeline. In general, your child will be in the hospital for at least 30 days. They then need to stay near the BMT hospital for an additional 30 to 60 days, depending on how they recover. The following sections cover things we found that pertain to BMT specifically.

Nathan's home hospital did not offer BMT. They worked with a larger hospital with a BMT team for the patients that needed a transplant. This other hospital has a very large BMT program with many staff members and patients. Our experiences below reflect this large BMT environment. Many of the sections below still apply even if your child's BMT is done at a smaller facility.

Treatment Overview

After frontline chemotherapy, your child's disease should be controlled, the bone marrow should be clear, and very little, if any, visible disease remaining. They call this minimal residual disease. Your child may also already be NED (meaning "no evidence of disease"). This is when the doctors can proceed to the intense chemotherapy called bone marrow transplant, or BMT. Very high dose "conditioning" chemotherapy is targeted to completely kill the remaining neuroblastoma cells but has the severe side effect of killing the bone marrow. To facilitate recovery, the stem cells harvested earlier are then given back to the child, so they can regrow their bone marrow.

The doctors follow the most current protocol with the best known detailed timeline for treatment and recovery. You should receive a copy of the protocol and have it on hand while in the hospital for your reference. If you have questions and there is not a medical staff member right there to help you, this is a good place to look for answers. There are too many details to try to remember.

In general, the treatment schedule looks like this:

- Your child receives a few days of intense chemotherapy
- Days later your child is injected with their own stem cells that were harvested earlier
- The intense side effects of mouth sores, pain, lethargy, etc., set in a couple days after stem cell infusion
- Wait until the stem cells engraft, grow, and begin producing white cells, red cells and platelets. This waiting and watching is the hardest part.
- Continue monitoring and care until strength returns

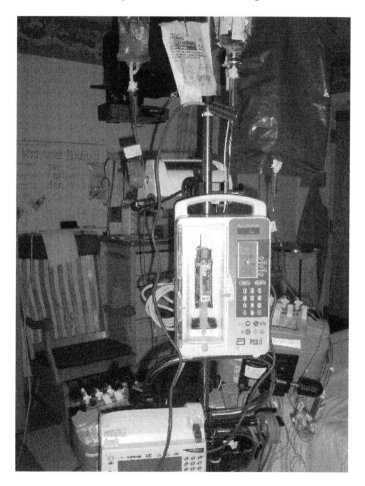

Figure 14 Nathan's very full BMT pole

This treatment is not like any seen to this point. The chemotherapy doses are very large and intense. The side effects can also be correspondingly bad and intense. Many of the palliative care measures used in the previous rounds of chemotherapy simply do not work. Your child will get more direct care from the nursing staff than ever before. During parts of this treatment, your child may keep a single nurse busy constantly. Even in the best scenario, this treatment will be a difficult time for you and your child. After the treatment is over and you have left the hospital, recovery can be long and slow. Your child is now considered immune compromised. You start to see the world differently. Wind will become a bad thing. You start to see germs everywhere: in the air ducts in your house, in the fallen leaves in the yard, in every sniffle and cough from a friend, and so on.

BMT Caregiver

Each day there will be visits by many staff members with a specific specialty and something they need to accomplish. Many of these come and go, doing their jobs without much input. The person who can help the most is your primary BMT caregiver, who in our case was a nurse practitioner. Again, we were in a large BMT facility. If BMT is done at a smaller hospital this may be your primary oncologist or some other medical staff member. They visit every morning before the doctor's rounds. Their job is to explain where you are in treatment and how things are going according to expectations for the treatment. BMT is done for many forms of cancer, not just neuroblastoma. Each cancer type has a different path through BMT.

The primary BMT caregiver usually explains the items to work on that day, whether it is trying to get your child to eat a bite or two of food or getting them up to walk. This is the point of contact that is constant throughout BMT. The doctors, nurses and other staff may rotate on and off as their schedules require, this BMT caregiver is usually the same for the 31 days of BMT and recovery. They work closely with the primary BMT oncologist as well as the staff "on service" and are the best way to get questions answered and concerns heard.

Every morning when our caregiver arrived at the room, we had a list of questions for him. *"Was Nathan doing ok?"* was usually the first. *"What should we try to do today?"*, *"Are you sure this is normal for BMT?"*, *"When can Kate come see him?"* were some of the others. Every morning he would answer any and all questions we had. *"Yes, Nathan is doing ok; he is following the expected steps through BMT."* *"You should keep Nathan happy, maybe get one or two sips of drink or food in him."* *"Yes, this is normal for BMT."* *"Kate can probably come see him in a few weeks."* He was always very patient and stayed with us as long as we needed him.

BMT Visitation

Limit visitation from friends and family in your child's hospital room. Every time a new person enters the room, they bring new germs to share with you and your child. Germs tend to hide on things like hands and shoes. Even if your visitor is not sick, they are carrying germs into the room. The medical staff is trained to reduce this risk, but your family and friends are not. Some family, like grandparents, or that special person that your child needs to see can come and be a big help to your child, but other family and friends should visit you someplace else. It could be the cafeteria or a lounge somewhere else in the hospital. Be very clear with your friends and family. It is not that they are not wanted; it is just not a good idea to introduce so many unknowns into such a controlled environment. The possibility of infection to you and your child is very great and very real. The flu now has the possibility of being fatal to your child. Infections of any sort can slow down or complicate recovery. The best way to protect your child is to keep visitors out of your child's room. For those you need to have there, make sure to find out the rules for visitations and follow them explicitly. Have them adequately trained, and then allow them to sit with your child so you can sleep a bit. You as the parent will have a very difficult time; just watching your child being this sick is exhausting. Realize early that you cannot do this on your own. It is not a good idea to even try. Whether your helpers are in the room or not, lean on them. Lean on your friends, family, church, and spouse. Allow family and friends to bring meals down to you at the hospital and spend time in the parents' lounge relaxing and eating with you.

We had three family members taking care of Nathan during our time at BMT: me, Scott, and Scott's mother. We set up a rotation of people to stay overnight at the hospital and to stay at home to care for Kate. Having that third person to help made a big difference to Scott and me but it especially made a difference to Kate. She was able to have a more stable home life through this time. We also had family and friends come to the hospital and bring us meals. A few came just to chat. This was quite the commitment since the hospital was a bit of a drive. We had a very strong support team behind us, and BMT was still very difficult on us all.

New Way to do Things

Many times BMT is not done at your "home hospital," and you may need to travel to a hospital that specializes in bone marrow transplants. The advantage to a larger BMT hospital is that the staff treats a lot of children just like yours each day. You are there for this expertise. The disadvantage may be that you are now working with a new team, a new set of doctors, nurses, and medical staff. We found this part a bit overwhelming. We learned to listen to the team, ask them questions as needed, work with them rather than against them, and do not argue at each decision because it is different than how we had done it in the past. You can look at it this way: these are the people who know BMT best, and you know your child the best. Working together is the obvious best solution.

In our case, I had difficulty remembering all the things I was told during our hours long discussions with the doctor while preparing to sign the consent forms. I found myself asking the same questions over and over and still not exactly remembering all of it, and they were only telling me the parts I needed to know. It was helpful to me to reread the consent forms and read over the treatment protocol. Most of the time, I was content to allow the staff to do their jobs and not try to take over and do it myself (not that I could). We knew they were there to help us and our family. We needed to let go of our anger for having to be there in the first place and not take it out on the staff. Sometimes we were more successful than others. It can be very frustrating being in BMT even when all things go well.

If BMT is at a new hospital there are many things to get familiar with: the new hospital layout, their standard protocols, and the staff. When you go to a new and sometimes bigger hospital, many things are a bit uncomfortable. That "home" feeling of your familiar hospital is not there. Do not let this affect how you care for your child. Make sure you take the experience you have gained during frontline chemotherapy to help the new staff learn about your child. It is very difficult going from a hospital where you are already comfortable with the staff, where you can discuss things easily with them, to a hospital that does things differently and you do not know any of the staff.

When Nathan went through his first rounds of chemotherapy, the team at our home hospital came up with very specific regimes of nausea and pain medicines that kept him mostly comfortable through treatment. As long as we kept to that schedule precisely, he fared reasonably well, with minimum vomiting and pain. When we got to the larger hospital for BMT, our regimen for pain and nausea was not standard for them. I had to discuss with the staff the methods that worked for Nathan earlier in treatment and see if they could accommodate his specific needs. It took a few "extra" conversations and a discussion with the pharmacist, but in the end they were able to work with our proven method and incorporate it into their plan. After a while even our home regime did not keep up with the nausea, but we had been able to keep Nathan comfortable longer using a regime that had been shown to work for him. There were many instances where the BMT staff did things differently than what we were used to, but most of the time these methods were just as effective.

One of the things I've learned through the whole journey is that doctors do things with a purpose in mind. Most things are not random or overlooked even though they may seem that way at first. For example, the BMT team takes your child's vitals frequently, let them. Do not complain that your child is getting his blood pressure done every hour during the night because it might wake him, usually it does not wake the child. It is very important that the doctors know if there is any change in your child vitals, specifically blood pressure. An elevated blood pressure can be a warning sign of a severe toxicity. A lower blood pressure may be a sign that your child has an infection. Look at it this way: a small child should not have an abnormal blood pressure under most circumstances, even during BMT. If your child does have an abnormal blood pressure, you should ask yourself why. Remember, you can always ask any question you need; if you want to know why something is being done to your child, ask. The staff can only address your question or concern if you voice it. Sitting in the room getting angry about something helps no one. Talk to the staff. Remember your and their goal is the get your child through BMT.

By the time your child starts BMT, they should be used to being in a hospital with people poking at them. Within reason they handle it fine. To illustrate, earlier at our home hospital, Nathan had to be admitted for fever. During the long visit at the ED and waiting in the room for the admitting resident, Nathan had fallen asleep since it was after midnight. The admitting resident came in and was complaining that he could not finish his assessment of Nathan without waking him. I asked the resident to try and ask Nathan to open his mouth and whatever else he needed while Nathan was still asleep. The resident asked Nathan to open his mouth, Nathan did as asked. Nathan never woke up and the resident was able to complete his assessment.

Every once in a while something "dopey" happens, where things just don't work as they should. Without malice or intent, something goes wrong. Don't hold on to these things. If something does happen, address it, resolve it, and then let it go. We have a whole list of "dopey" events that happened throughout Nathan's care at hospitals. Dwelling on them after they are resolved does nothing for anyone either. Nathan does not remember any of them.

During BMT, there may be times when things don't go, what you would consider, smoothly. That is simply the nature of BMT. BMT therapy is much harsher than the first rounds of chemotherapy. Even if your child gets through BMT in a relatively straight forward way, it may still seem horrible to you. Most times the treatments arrive and are delivered as you discussed with the doctor, sometimes they are not. Things can change quickly during BMT; doctors might give instructions for a therapy before they have time to discuss it with the family. Being fast sometimes is a key to saving lives. Doctors on the BMT floor are attending many families at once. It is unreasonable for them to hold up a therapy just because they did not discuss it with the family first. If you watch the BMT staff doing their work, you will see they are constantly busy. Most times, the nurses on the BMT floor have a single patient, sometimes two. These people never stop moving or working for their entire shift, and they only have one or two children to work with. The effort and dedication of the staff can be seen clearly if you look. BMT treatment is harsh, things can happen and happen quickly, and there is little as a parent you can do about it other than hug your child, read to your child, and comfort your child.

BMT Oncologist

Going into BMT, you work with a primary BMT oncologist. This is the doctor from whom you should learn everything you need to know about the treatment. It is easy to forget most of this information since it is quite complex and very foreign to most people. Try to focus on the parts that you need to know and make notes in your journal about the parts on which you may want more information. Your primary BMT oncologist is the one you follow up with after leaving the hospital while staying nearby the BMT hospital until your child is cleared to return to their home hospital. Know how to contact your primary BMT oncologist. Get their email or phone number and ask them when it is appropriate to contact them. On at least one occasion during Nathan's time on BMT, she was able to answer a question quickly and resolve one of those "dopey" incidents.

If in a large BMT hospital, your primary BMT oncologist may not be the doctor you see every day while staying in the hospital. Doctors take turns being "on service," covering the patients admitted for treatment. The on service doctor is the person you work with for your child's day to day care while in patient on BMT. They will answer your questions and discuss daily activities. These doctors usually change every week or two. During your stay for BMT, you can have four or more doctors taking care of your child. Some of these doctors you connect with immediately and work well with. Others you will not. Make sure you allow the working relationship to take priority regardless of how well you get along with them. Also, for extreme circumstances, have a way to contact your primary BMT oncologist in case you need clarification on something that happened.

Things You Cannot Control During BMT

Journal entry–" His numbers are still zero and he is still miserable, but as the doctors have told us, "Just get to the other side," and that is what we are doing."

BMT is the most intense treatment and attention received during frontline therapy. There will be many doctors, nurses, and other staff caring for your child. These people are experts in the field and work with BMT patients all day every day. For your child's good, you may have very little control over most of the medical things during BMT; I recommend you don't even try. You will hear many new medical terms, see new scans and, learn many new horrible things that may happen to your child. Do not spend your time worrying about these things; spend your time trying to make your child as comfortable as possible. Spend your time reading to them, snuggling with them, watching TV with them, or telling stories to them, anything to distract them from what they are going through. This can be a tough time for parents. You will probably see your child sicker than ever before. Your child's appearance can change with the effects of the chemotherapy, and you may feel helpless. You need to stay focused on those few things you can control, such as being positive around your child, paying attention to what the staff tells you, following the instructions as best you can, and being as helpful as possible.

Journal entry– "Today was the first day of bad."

Our good memories of BMT are of the families we met. We ran into them in the parents' lounge, cafeteria, or gift shop. We would talk with them, share with them, and allow them to comfort us. We still keep in touch with some of them. We would inevitable discuss treatments, histories, plans, and all things medical. I would like to put in a bit of caution when talking with other neuroblastoma families. Remember all the children have gotten to BMT down a different road, with different symptoms, different stages of disease, different diagnoses, and different treatments and protocols. Just remember, every child has their own treatment plan and just because another child is doing something different than yours, do not get worried that perhaps their path is better.

Journal entry- "Up until now, whenever I arrive at the hospital Nathan would usually hunt through my back pack to see what cool toys and things I had brought for him. He would stop all conversation until my back pack was COMPLETELY emptied and checked a few times, then he would continue on his way (he loves getting stuff no matter how small, he's four, go figure). Now for the perspective: Nathan has three boxes, one package and one card that sit unopened on the floor beside his BMT bed. He just doesn't feel well enough to care about them yet. Oh he will, and we will tear through them, but we are just not there yet."

Things You Can Control During BMT

There are a few things you do have some control over during BMT. Mostly these are comfort things for your child.

Pain

Your child may have a lot of pain due to side effects and the severity of the chemotherapy. Many hospitals have a pain management team. During BMT they should visit daily and discuss the options you have at your disposal. They are the ones who will make sure your child gets the right amount of pain medicine and not too much. Work with the pain team to give your child whatever medicine you need to help him through this treatment. We chose to give Nathan as much pain medicine as possible so that he would sleep as many hours as possible in a day. Nathan slept for 20 hours most days. The pain team said they could pull back a bit on the pump so he would be awake more; my response was whether they could increase the medicine so he would sleep even more. *"Just get to the other side."*

Comfort

The few hours a day Nathan was awake we would do anything to make him any bit happier. If there is any position for your child that is comfortable, use it, even if it is them lying on your chest for hours. One day Nathan decided that the only way he was going to sleep soundly was on my chest. He slept there for hours. When I left he would sleep on Scott. When I returned the next day Scott and I switched again. When Grandma was there, Nathan slept next to her. It was one of the few times we felt like we were really helping him.

Another one of Nathan's favorite activities was listening to books, and is still a favorite activity to this day. We found an online library that actually read kid's books out loud. Nathan does not remember any of his time on BMT but he does remember many of these books. Nathan would lie there mostly unconscious, but I had books playing all the time. One of his favorites was about the tooth fairy. When he lost his first tooth years later, this book came back to him. He informed me all about the tooth fairy and how she would act, where she came from, and what she would do with the teeth, all from this book.

Again, every child is different. We met kids that worked through BMT with video games. Others loved massages. Others watched TV. Find what works and use it, over and over and over and over, until your child wants something else. Then do that.

Feeding Tube

When mouth sores develop on BMT they are more severe than any you have seen so far. They start in the mouth and end at the bottom. When your child feels this horrible, they stop eating and drinking. All things that enter the mouth, medicine, food, and drinks, hurt. There are some medicines that can only be given by mouth. These pose a tough problem with severe mouth sores. Mouth sores can be bypassed by using a feeding tube, which is a small tube that goes up through the nose and down the esophagus into the stomach. There are many benefits to having a feeding tube. It helps deliver food and medicine directly to the stomach, bypassing the terrible mouth sores. If you use a feeding tube you need to put it in before the mouth sores start, otherwise the insertion of the feeding tube would cause more trouble than it would help.

The major drawback is that your child might not want one; your child may be scared of the procedure and having something new. They are scared about most everything at this point. You as the parent can probably find a positive way to present the feeding tube option to your child. You can use very creative solutions like, "*You can get your medications without me waking you up or tasting the meds you don't like,*" or "*It will help you eat and get better sooner so you can play with your sister*". With Nathan I probably just needed to bribe him with a stuffed cat.

Nathan did NOT want one, he was completely against it and therefore we did not push him. Again, I'm not sure if this was the best course of action, but it is the one we took. In hind sight, it sure would have been wonderful to see him eat something sooner than he did. That would have been an indescribable help. Talk with the doctor and primary BMT caregiver to weigh your options in regards to a feeding tube.

Using the Facilities

Your child will most likely lose any control over their bowels. Many times they cannot get up and go to the bathroom without severe pain. Other times the bowel movements are just liquid and they simply cannot control them. There can be many accidents, where the bed linens need to be changed a few times a day. They are not eating any food or drinking. All fluids are intravenous. They have just had the most intense chemotherapy they will see and they are sleeping all day. Messy bowels should not be a surprise. The solution may be as simple as a diaper. This sounds easy enough, but in their weakened condition it may be something they just don't want. You may be able to find a way to convince them to use some form of diaper if they are not already in one. You can let them know how wonderful they are and this is just to help them sleep. In our case, cleaning up after Nathan was not a problem for us or the hospital staff; it was a problem for Nathan. He felt so hurt because, as a big boy of four years old, he should be able to control this. I very gently asked if he wanted a diaper so that he did not have these accidents. *Nope, diapers are for babies.* A day later I asked the same question about pull-up diapers that had a picture of a much older boy on the package. This time he accepted. He still had to get up when we changed his pull-up, but now it was on his terms and he was in control of the one thing he could control.

A Little Bit of Recovery

Eventually your child's Absolute Neutrophil Count, ANC, starts to recover. There will be a nonzero ANC one day, a small blip. The next day it may go back to zero. And finally it starts to steadily climb. The primary BMT caregiver told us a couple days early to let us know this was coming. We did not believe him. He was right. He also told us that Nathan would be leaving the hospital about 10 days later. We did not believe him then either. This time he was only one day off. We left 11 days later.

Once your child's ANC starts climbing, many of the more severe side effects start going away. Your child's mouth sores become less severe, the heart rate goes back to a normal pace, the lethargy starts to go away (especially with the help of a little sister), and they want to start doing little kid things again. Eventually, you get to leave the hospital and go back home.

As Nathan started recovering from BMT, he was allowed a couple "outings" in the hospital where he was able to leave his room and walk around. At this time Nathan's favorite toy was his Nerf Long Shot gun. The room was way too small for him to shoot it in the room without hurting one of us. He asked the doctor, very politely, if he could shoot it down the hallway. There, he and Scott laid on a blanket on the floor on one end of the hallway and tried to shoot the window down at the other end. The funniest part of the game was the nurses, staff, parents, and patients going in and coming out of the rooms with no notice. Scott reported that *no passers-by were injured, although one startled woman may have had a small accident.* This event completely wiped Nathan out, and he slept for the next several hours with a big smile on his face.

Nathan was finishing up his BMT treatment. His ANC was increasing, his mouth sores and other symptoms were going away, but our happy little boy was not back yet. He was listless, lethargic, and blah. We talked with Nathan's primary BMT doctor about Nathan's sister Kate coming to visit since kids less than seven years old were not allowed on the BMT floor at our hospital.

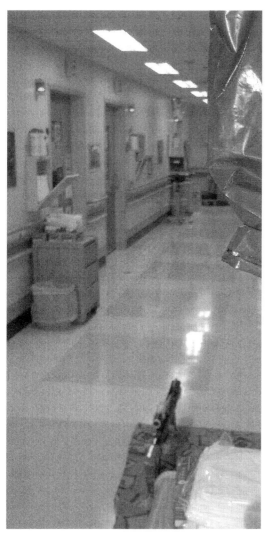

Figure 15 Nathan and Scott's first post BMT outing

Kate was two at the time. The doctors decided it would be safe and we received special permission for her visit. When she got there, Nathan was just lying in bed staring blankly at the TV. Kate came over, climbed into bed with him and took his blanket. She then requested (demanded) that he watch Little Einsteins (HER favorite show). Nathan turned the channel for her. Kate started to chatter at him. Nathan started to smile. A little bit into the show, the Little Einsteins said *"Pat, pat, pat, Blast off"*. By this point Nathan had a big smile, had his arms in the air with Kate, and was yelling at the top of his lungs, *"BLAST OFF"*. At that moment, our happy little boy returned for good. We knew then, thanks to his sister, Kate, that he was going to be just fine.

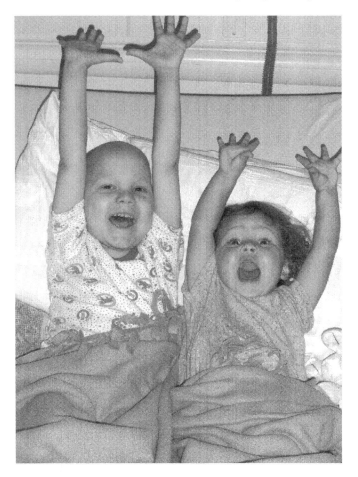

Figure 16 Pat, Pat, Pat, BLAST OFF!

Leaving the Hospital

One thing that came with Nathan's starting to feel better was attitude. Once he was not sleeping 20 hours a day, he felt just fine letting us know what he wanted and when. The biggest thing for him was that he wanted to leave the hospital. That was the first question every morning, "*When can we go home?*" and the last one at night, "*Can we go home tomorrow?*" Do not rush leaving the hospital. When your child is ready, the staff will let you leave the hospital. This is one area where patience is very difficult but very important. It might be difficult staying in the hospital for more than a month, but it is best to let the BMT staff decide when it is time to go home. Nathan decided that it was his primary BMT oncologist's fault that he was still in the hospital. She started receiving his attitude. He ignored her whenever she came into the room. He would not even pretend he was sleeping, he was just mad at this person; it was their fault. Finally, the time came that we were discussing leaving the hospital. Nathan's doctor entered the room, Nathan ignored her, and then she mentioned that he had to talk to her before she would let him leave. That was all the convincing he needed. His head spun to her and a big smile came over his face. His charm now was directed at only one person, and she was going to let him leave.

The biggest thing about moving out of the hospital after a month of BMT is that now YOU need to know how to care for your child. A lot of things are going on constantly during treatment while you are in the hospital. Now you need to learn how to do all those things. You will be trained, but once you are out of the hospital, you will need to handle it all. Scott describes it perfectly in this journal entry.

Journal entry– "Well, after spending the final 2 days at the hospital, I let Rachel and Grandma go home and I took the first 2 days at Ronald McDonald House. This is actual work. Did you know there are no nurses here? Well, except Grandma, and we let her go home once in a while. The kid is taking 7 oral medications...some 3 times a day, some every 8 hours (no those aren't the same), some twice a day, some once a day, and some as needed...plus 2 IV medications...and gets IV nutrition for 12 hours at night which involves testing his...yes...urine for sugar and ketones (nothing to do with music). Luckily, it is not a taste test. Anyway, it's a good thing the women in my life got the system set up for me beforehand. Otherwise, I would be lost." – Scott

Ronald McDonald House

After leaving the hospital, BMT follow up care usually requires daily or every other day visits to the hospital for a few weeks depending on how quickly your child recovers. If the hospital is a long distance from your home it would be helpful to stay in a facility near the hospital. There are a couple organizations that can help: the Ronald McDonald House (RMH) and the Fisher House to name a couple. We stayed at the Ronald McDonald House next to the hospital after BMT. The Ronald McDonald House is an amazing organization. They give and care constantly for the families in their house. Meals are brought in by volunteers. They are quiet and very well organized. They have outings for families in their care. And on special occasions they have parties for the guests. The hospital social worker assisted us in getting a room when we needed it. BMT patients had special care instructions and rooms at the RMH. We know of at least one RMH that is just for childhood cancer patients.

Total Parenteral Nutrition

After the worst side effects of BMT start going away, your child might not be eating or drinking much of anything. The mouth sores and other stress on the body during the entire process takes a huge toll on their system. They may simply not be interested in eating or drinking, and who could blame them? If this is the case, the doctor might put them on a nutritional aid called total parenteral nutrition or TPN. TPN has nutrients and glucose for the system to keep it going until they are able to eat again. TPN is usually given during sleeping hours. It is only a short term solution, but it helps your child until they start eating again on their own. TPN cannot be done indefinitely without hurting internal organs. The best way to stop using TPN is to get your child to start eating.

Eating

Journal entry– *"So far so good. Nathan is feeling as expected. His throat hurts, he is nauseous, and he is weak. Considering all that he has been through, he's in pretty good spirits. He even continues to postpone bedtime with the usual ploys "Mommy, I didn't get a bed time snack". Now the boy gagged on his mouthwash and was now asking for food, so I took advantage of him. I got a Frito chip and 5 cheerios in him. That is a big success in my book."*

Nathan did not eat for weeks. He did not eat anything at all even after the mouth sores went away. We were constantly trying to get him to eat something, bribery did not work, ordering him never worked, enticing him with his favorite food did not help. To help his appetite, we started him on an appetite stimulant that he had taken in the past, hoping it would help him overcome the memory of the mouth sores. We knew that he had to get over this as soon as he could; he was getting too skinny for our tastes. We never gave up. We never got angry at Nathan, though we may have gotten frustrated at our inability to help him eat. We did get creative in our attempts. Scott had dad methods to entice him, I had mom methods. We just kept trying anything we could think of.

For the first few weeks after leaving the hospital, we stayed at the Ronald McDonald House. Many wonderful people bring meals in for those staying at the house. One night a church group brought in a hotdog bar with all the fixings. I made myself two hotdogs with cheese on them and a salad. When I returned to the room, Nathan started to eye my food. He had not yet been interested in food, so I was very excited about this. He finally asked me *"Mom, may I please have that?"* With a smile on my face I handed him my hotdog with cheese. He took the hotdog off the bun placed it on my plate and proceeded to eat the bun and cheese. SUCCESS! He was eating again. That was the start of his cheese and starch menu for months. He would eat cheese with most things, macaroni and cheese, bread and cheese, even just slices of American cheese. Scott got very creative in his way to give Nathan cheese and bread. Meals went from getting Nathan to eat anything to an exercise of putting as many calories as possible into him. Any food works, Nathan just happened upon cheese and bread.

Intravenous Immunoglobulin

Your child's immune system is "suppressed" with the newly engrafted bone marrow. Their bodies do not have the strength to fight off any germs at first. The immune system takes a long time to recover, at least a year or more before the severe restrictions are lifted. In order to help recovery, they might be given intravenous immunoglobulin (IVIG). IVIG is a blood product, rich in antibodies, that recognizes and helps fight certain infections. It is giving back antibodies to your child so that they have some form of defense against germs. IVIG is administered by IV in four different rate levels. The level is increased after a short period of time. Initially IVIG is administered weekly, after a bit, it goes to every other week, then monthly, until their system shows enough improvement that they can stop it completely.

As with any blood product, there can be an adverse reaction. Look for signs and keep a close eye on your child while the IVIG is being administered. For example, their heart rate can soar, they can get glossy eyed, and they can go into convulsions. As with the other blood products, there are things that can be done to resolve the issue the next time your child gets the product, such as premedicating and not administering it at the problematic rate level. Nathan had such a reaction. During one IVIG treatment, Nathan started having convulsions and his heart rate soared. I freaked out and called the nurse. She reduced the administrated rate and the symptoms went away. For the remaining IVIG treatments, we just kept the rate low enough and Nathan was able to receive them without incident.

Physical Therapy

Your child will probably be physically very weak after the treatment and inactivity while they were feeling so crummy. They may have difficulty standing on their own. They may not be able to walk and may need a wheelchair. Be ready for this. Be patient and help your child as they recover their strength and stamina. In many hospitals there is a formal Physical Therapy (PT) program available for your child as they recover. I recommend using PT to help your child take their first steps to recovery. The physical therapist can help with the BMT specific issues. They know the exact muscles to use to get the most benefit to help recovery. However, physical therapy does not always need to be formalized with a therapist. PT can be getting down on the floor playing games, moving around, bearing their own weight, hitting a ball, or playing golf. Any kid playing activity that requires movement is a form of physical therapy.

Nathan had a lot of trouble getting around after BMT. He could not stand for very long and could hardly walk except very short distances. He had issues with his right leg being slightly turned in towards his left leg. There was no way he could have run. We felt over time this would improve, but it was very heart breaking watching him get so winded with such minimal excursions. We tried to address Nathan's physical weaknesses slowly and with as much patience and toughness as we could. Nathan was offered physical therapy treatment while we were in the hospital and at the Ronald McDonald House. These sessions were very helpful, but they were short and only once a day. Nathan had his own form of PT when recovering at the Ronald McDonald House. He would pick up a large blow up dinosaur and charge at Scott. They would race back and forth until he was so out of breath he could not run anymore. Then the boys would collapse and laugh.

Once Back Home

Finally, it is time to get back home in normal surroundings. Be ready, there is a big difference from when you last left for the hospital with your child for BMT. It has been months since your child has been home, and your child is a different person now. They are very weak and very susceptible to any germ or virus. They bruise easily and take a very long time to heal. Remember, your child's immune system is brand new and does not know how to fight off anything. None of the vaccines they got as a baby still work. Any virus they have already had and beaten can come back (Nathan has had the chicken pox 3 times and H1N1 3 times). Your BMT oncologist should have a list of recommendations for your house before your child returns home and a list of things your child can and cannot do once there. Their immune system may be weaker now than when they were new born, which is a good way to think about it. Treat your child more carefully than when they were first born.

Many of the precautions are intuitive, such as washing hands when you come into the house, having no sick visitors, being very alert for fevers, and so on. We even put up signs at every door requesting hand washing upon entering. Other precautions made

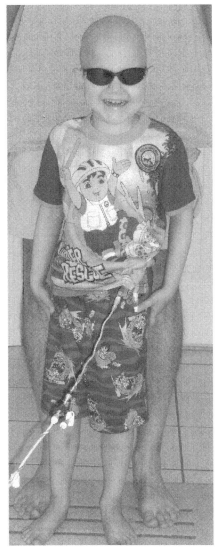

Figure 17 Back home after BMT

sense upon reflection, there was more worry of the fish tank being one large bacteria colony than there was with the dog. You wash your hands after touching the dog, no licking the face and so on. You do not touch the fish tank. We learned how many different filters you can put on a heating system to remove the most amounts of contaminants. We had the air ducts and carpets cleaned. Can you remember the last time that was done?

Your medical team will give you specific instructions to follow when the time comes, here is a brief list of some of our go home instructions:

Visitors
- For the first month he should be treated as if he is still in the hospital.
- Not visiting if they have been sick in the past week
- No kissing, just waving
- Keep most people 3 feet away

Outside
- You care about dirt, dust, and mold
- Only go out on clean, calm days when it is not too dusty
- No swinging
- No digging in the dirt
- No windy days
- No group settings, no church, no mall, no movies, nothing with a large group.
- If eating out, only have fresh cooked food that is still hot and has not been under a warmer
- Don't feed the dog
- Wash hands after petting the dog
- No cleaning
- Keep him out of a house for at least an hour after the house is finished being cleaned
- Stay away from bird droppings
- Wash towels and anything that absorbs fluids once a week
- Change the dish wash rag or sponge daily

- Play at your house, not friends' houses. You know how clean your house is.

We found even more amazing people after Nathan went home. Our home heat pump broke during the coldest week of winter. It had to be replaced and quickly. We did the usual research and getting estimates, but this time we had a few extra requirements, specifically their best air purifiers for Nathan. We would briefly mention why we needed one and then ask for a quote. The third quote we got was for the best HVAC system available with the best air purifier on the market. It was way out of our price range but would be the best for Nathan. The next day I got a message on our answering machine. The manager from CJS Heating and Air called us back and said that he had spent the entire evening thinking about Nathan and how CJS could help. He said, if we chose his company, he would love to install the UV air purifying system for us for free. And, if we DID NOT choose his company, he wanted to leave the UV air purifier system on our door step so that the other company could install it. He just "wanted to do this." We, of course, chose them for the whole project.

Final BMT Thoughts

BMT is a long hard treatment. There are a lot of tough things that happen during this treatment. Some days seem like a crisis. Other days seem like they last forever. In the end, your child is hopefully free of neuroblastoma. This is a tough treatment, take it seriously and don't take it personally. The best part of BMT is that Nathan remembers none of it.

NOTES

NOTES

NOTES

CHAPTER 5. HOW TO MANAGE CANCER 101

There were many non-medical things that we learned in our family's journey. Some may seem obvious while others are less apparent until you read it or see it done. The following sections are by no means inclusive; however, they are the key things Scott and I would like to share.

You Cannot Cure Cancer

As a parent, we were completely overwhelmed with our new reality of cancer. We went into "fix it" mode. How do we cure this cancer? How do we fix this problem? Where do we start? How do we get things to go back to normal? You, the mom or dad, cannot cure cancer. Do not waste all your time trying. Sometimes the doctors cannot cure cancer. Please research your child's type of treatment but don't do it to the distraction of your real need, caring for your child. It is important to have knowledge of what treatments are available and where. It is more important that you do not allow this to be total focus of your attention. There are many things you can spend your time doing to help your child.

Online Blogs

Trying to keep all the family, friends and neighbors and their family and friends current on everything that is going on can be a daunting task. First, who wants to retell the daily events over and over and over to each loving person? It was hard the first time. There is email, but it is also very tough to include everyone on an email chain (trust me; we had over 200 on our distribution list). The solution is online blogs.

There are three free online blogs that we know of. These are designed to help keep people informed. They are Caringbridge.org, Carepages.org, and recently Colespages.org. These sites let you keep a running blog about your child's care. The websites notify people of a new entry and allow them to go get it themselves without your help.

You can put in photos, let your child choose their own style, and friends can leave messages and prayers. A friend of ours started Nathan's Caringbridge site. She chose Caringbridge, created the site and would up load our emails to the blog whenever we sent one out. It was a very sweet thing for her to do while we were overwhelmed with all the other things taking our attention. Eventually, we started managing the site ourselves. Each night before bed we would allow a few moments to relive the day and put down the points that would be interesting to family and friends. It became very therapeutic. When Nathan became aware of the site he would have us read the entries to him and ask to add things that he felt we had missed. We, of course, did not read to him all the medical stuff, just the kid stuff. Nathan also enjoyed hearing all the messages left for him. At three years old he was not a reader, so he loved it when he could listen to the stories friends would tell.

When we started writing the Caringbridge website ourselves, we found it strange. Writing on a blog was new to us. I did not know how public these sites were. Who would read them? What if the doctor or nurses were to read it? What if we got the information wrong and started more problems than we helped? How could someone put all these feeling, tests, scans and other technical and personal information in a blog for all to see? Should we use the doctors and nurses names? Were we even allowed to? In the end we treated the blog like a letter to a friend. We did not use it as a diary or as a timeline of events that we may or may not have heard correctly (remember only 10% memory on tough subjects). We would write stories about Nathan and how he was feeling. We would write how wonderful the people around us were and how they would go out of their way to do crazy things in order to make Nathan smile. We would write down personal feelings because sometimes you just need to let them out. We would write down the scans, tests, and key events that were coming up. We tended to include any positive information we could and tried to avoid just whining and complaining, even though it is very easy to do. We would put on photos of that amazing boy so that all could share what we see in him, even photos of him taking a bath in a pink bucket. Nathan's Caringbridge site is the foundation for most of the information in this book.

One of the most interesting powers of Nathan's Caringbridge site was how it made things he wanted materialize out of thin air. On occasion he would ask to include random things on his blog, things that he wanted. Orange golf clubs was the most interesting one. It NEVER failed that within a few days these items would just materialize on our front porch and he would get to play with them. He felt he had very great power and still does not really grasp that you have to buy things; they don't just appear.

Here is a sample Caringbridge.org entry:

TUESDAY, AUGUST 15

Hi All,

Nathan is going along pretty much at the same pace. He is hot and cold, sweating and dry, omery and mousey, playful and quiet. Since he cannot get down to play in the fort to get away from the doctors, today he decided to pretend he was asleep to get away from them. It would have worked better if he did not answer all their questions and open his mouth when asked to. The doctors and nurses cracked up.

He did get up for a walk. More of those will help in his recovery. He did get a bath even though he was fighting it. And he does feel better. We have gotten into our routine which is good for all and good to not look long term too much. Katie is doing just fine. She is playing with Daddy right now.

A friend of ours got Nathan duty today. Later, I will send some awesome pictures of the kids that she took today.

God Bless,

Rachel

Bribery

It is a common challenge for parents to find ways to get their child to allow the doctors to perform the required scans, tests and labs. This is an ongoing endeavor many times a week. We tried many tactics, but we have been pleasantly surprised how well bribery worked on our son. He gets poked, prodded, scanned, and drugged - you name it - and he does most anything for a small toy or trip to the gift shop. We are happy when the scan, or test, or treatment gets completed without us having to physically restrain him. He is happy when he gets to leave the room to shop and gets to play with the new toy.

Over the years the bribery items changes. It started as stuffed cats and has moved on to apps for his tablet. It is truly amazing how well Nathan behaves for a $0.99 app.

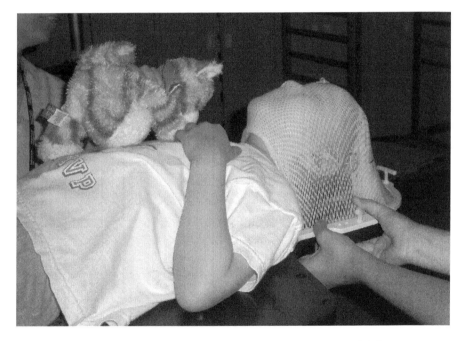

Figure 18 Nathan prepping for radiation treatment with his newest bribery item, a stuffed cat

Journal entry – *"My son did show me how well he can manipulate me today. While getting fitted for hearing aids he threw a COMPLETE fit about getting stuff stuck in his ears. Mind you we had been at the hospital for five hours or so by then. We tried bribing him and threatening him, but what finally worked was the video Rocky and Bullwinkle. When he was all done, boy did he rein in all those bribes that were offered at the front. He had a big smile on his face by this point. He is sure a cutie."*

A Long Road

Childhood cancer treatment is a hard thing to visualize when you are just starting the journey. You cannot imagine that it will probably completely consume at least one parent in the household for years. It takes a LONG time and, even when it is over, you still have to deal with the long term side effects. Eventually you come to the realization that you most likely will not have your normal life back. All your life's perspective and priorities get changed for good. The following sections touch on some of these areas.

Not Your Fault

The first thing to realize is that it is NOT your fault that your child has cancer. I'm sure in some rare cases it is hereditary, but, in general, your actions did not give your child cancer. I have to admit I had a lot of trouble with this topic. I did believe that it was my fault that Nathan got cancer. He was knitted in my womb. I believed that while in my body something went wrong in his body as I put him together. In reality, I'm sure there is nothing I did specifically that gave him cancer, and probably there was nothing I could have done differently during pregnancy to prevent him from getting it. I truly understand how hard it is to come to grip with this reality; I have a very hard time not blaming myself.

This manifested itself into a very big problem for me the first three or so months after diagnosis. The absolute worst thing for me was changing Nathan's central line dressing. He would scream and yell because the tape hurt when it came off. I would cry and cry because this was my precious little boy with a tube sticking out of his chest and it was my fault. This sweet little thing had cancer and I gave it to him. It was not the act of taking the bandage off that was horrific, even though it was bad; it was the fact that every time I did it I saw the dreaded disease eating away at this gift from God. I did eventually work through this self-blame, mostly. To tell you the truth, it was Nathan that helped me. This three year old boy would no longer let me feel sorry for him; he and I were going to figure out how to get that darn bandage off without causing so much pain and without leaving his skin red and irritated. So started our love for alcohol wipes. We would soak that tape and take it off one very small spot at a time. We had all the time we needed. We made sure we were never in a rush. Over time, he got less sensitive and I got more liberal with the wipes, and we made it through the year with a Broviac central line. Our lesson from this is that it does no good to dwell on why your child has cancer. Instead, spend this time with your child who happens to have cancer.

Not God's Fault

I have met people who blame God for their child's cancer. He is a good candidate for the blame. He is big enough, He can handle it; however, it is not God's fault. He did not zap your child and give them cancer; I don't think He works that way. It is just the world we live in, sometimes crappy things happen. The bigger question is what you will do about it?

Here is a story I remember from church:

One day there was this terrible flood. A devout man prayed to be saved by God. He had climbed onto his roof and was waiting for God to rescue him. A row boat came by. The man in the boat offered to take the devout man to safety. He said, "No, God will rescue me". A little while later, after more prayer, a motor boat came up and offered a ride to safety. The devout man again refused, saying that God was going to rescue him. After more prayer a helicopter flew by and offered to rescue the man. He refused one final time saying that God would rescue him. In the end the man drowned. Standing at the doors of heaven the man asked God why he had not saved him. God replied "I sent you a row boat, when that failed I sent you a motor boat, when that failed I sent you a helicopter."

To continue with this analogy, I see the row boat as the medical staff, doctors, nurses, etc. They are your front line, your first rescue, your biggest advocates and helpers. You see them daily, you get to know them and care for them. Your child will most likely be on a first name basis with almost everyone at the hospital. With their help, your child will get the best treatment possible. Let them care for you and your family. Rely on their strength and expertise. When you have a question or concern, ask someone. They have all done this before; they are there for your family and your child.

I see the motor boat as your friends, family, church, and neighbors. We had amazing help through our journey. Our friends and neighbors did not know how to cure cancer, but they sure knew how to keep our yard in shape. They knew how to come play with the kids when we were home so that Scott and I could get some sleep. We rarely asked for anything yet we had food, our home was cared for, our kids were loved, and our lives continued.

And, finally, the helicopter is the other families you meet on your journey. You spend many days with other kids with cancer and their families. Some have the same cancer as your child. Others have something you have never heard of and cannot pronounce. These will be the people God will speak through to you.

Hospital staff

I don't think it is possible to capture how amazing the medical staffs at the hospitals have been to our son and our family. From the first moment we entered the Hematology/Oncology department, our view of hospitals and their staffs changed forever. We have countless stories of their love and compassion while treating children with cancer. We have asked the same question over and over to the same person until we understood. In each case, they would sit with us, write it down, draw pictures, and do whatever it took until we understood it. Then they would do it again the next time we asked the same question. When it came to Nathan, they were truly angels. They sometimes went way beyond doing their jobs. On a few occasions, the cafeteria did not have that one food Nathan was willing to eat, so someone went and got it from the store.

The most compelling story was one we witnessed but were not involved in. While admitted on the Hematology/Oncology floor we met a little baby. She was a few months old, maybe a year. She had some rare form of cancer for which there was no treatment plan. No one knew how to even treat this child's disease. Her parents were very young and did the best they could. The hospital staff did not let this affect their care for this child. They would be in that room day after day snuggling that baby, cooing with that baby, caring for that baby, all the while knowing that their hearts were going to be broken.

Yes, there may be times when you run into care givers that are in a hurry, or don't talk to you very much or seem not to care. That can happen. The staff members have a hard job and I'm sure it gets to them sometimes, especially if things are going poorly. Try not to dwell on those moments. Rather, on those occasions, give some of that caring back to them. Nathan was excellent at cheering up staff members. If someone would come into the room a bit mopey, he would shoot them with a Nerf dart until they shot back, or he would ask them to snuggle, or he would just talk and giggle with them. He was a good example for us to follow.

Friends and Family

The biggest blessing we had during Nathan's cancer treatment was our friends and family. They came together in a way we could never have imagined. And they stayed. They didn't give up a few months into treatment; they kept on giving. They never got bored with story after story of how hard it was on Nathan, how the treatments were brutal, how tired we all were, how worried we were about Nathan and Kate, and so on. They just kept being there.

Scott's mother was our daily blessing for many months. She took a leave of absence from her work and moved in with us for 10 months through the worst of the treatment timeline. Many families we met were able to send their other children to grandparents for BMT. Not us, we moved the grandmother in. She had the added blessing of being a nurse and was perfectly comfortable in the world of medicine.

Many times we had family and friends arrive in town to help. They would show up in the waiting room for big events like surgery. The closest relative lived a 3 ½ hour drive way.

My sister called. *"When do you want me there?"* she asked. *"Tomorrow?!"* I replied. She was there.

Scott's folks and brother's family did not ask if they should come for surgery, the just came. My uncle did not ask what to do about orange golf clubs. Left handed youth golf clubs and a can of orange paint just appeared.

For the first few months, when we got home from the hospital there was something on the front step, every day. There were toys for the kids, there was food for us, there were letters, there were notes that "we just stopped by". There were endless concerns and mementos of love for our entire family. And it just kept coming.

The family we knew for years that took over most of Kate's care for the first many months until we got her into a daycare. We did not hear complaints about it from anyone but Kate.

The neighbors would gather in the street to discuss how to help without bothering us.

The church youth group adopted our family for Christmas after I said *"No, thank you"*. The same group purchased EVERYTHING on the list and then some so my kids had the most spectacular celebration that year.

The little friends that came over and treated Nathan like a kid, whether it was jumping on the beds or snuggling on the couch when he was too tired to move.

The friends that would show up in the hospital just to say, *"Hi"*. We had friends who did not want to bother us at the hospital, so they would leave notes or presents at the front desk, just so we knew they were thinking of us.

The different groups we knew who worked together with no help from us to organize meals and outings and babysitting and activities for the kids.

The occasional grandparent that kicked me and Scott out of the hospital to go have a meal together.

The friend that set up our on line blog and kept it updated with any information we gave her until we were able to take it over ourselves.

The volleyball Bible study group that continually cared for us spiritually and physically. They came over one day after I had a minor surgery to tackle our yard, gutters, and leaves.

The trips to Panera Bread with a friend just to let me vent, time and time again.

The sisters who knew that just two days away from it all, walking on the beach, would make such a difference, and so they made it happen, complete makeover included.

Scott's work gave him all the time off he needed, visited at the hospital, and threw parties for Nathan.

Our niece put her life on hold when we were in town for Nathan's treatment. She would see Nathan's dinosaurs as many times as he wanted and still acted thrilled by each visit. She made so many chicken nugget runs just because anticipating the yummy nuggets made treatment a tiny bit easier. She made a last minute run around the city to put together the best birthday Nathan could have. She was so affected by Nathan's life that she completely changed her career, and she now helps others dealing with cancer.

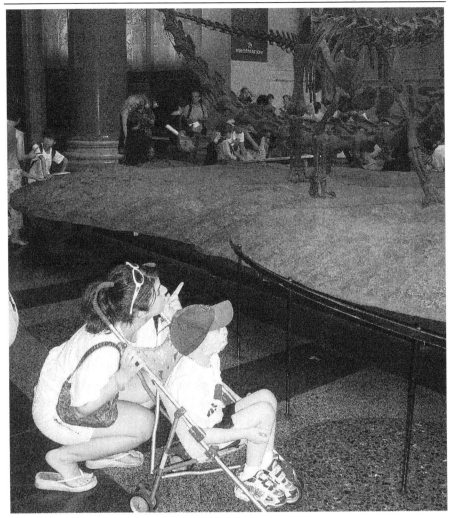

Our next door neighbors never asked to help us, they just did. Every week they knew I planned on using Saturday morning to do my yard work. Every week the yard was done on Thursday.

Our neighbor's daughter had returned home after college and had become a librarian in our area. She became one of Nathan's favorite people. Whenever we got home from the hospital his first question was always, "*Can I go see Jenna now?*" Jenna wrote about her time with Nathan for a story contest, I received a copy. Jenna (then 21) said I am welcome to share it here.

Bug Spray, Banquets and Blessings

By Jenna Bolles

The first time I met him, all I saw initially was one blinking brown eye. Our doorbell rang and through the tempered glass I saw a small person peering inside. Mildly irritated, but a little curious, I opened the door to find him standing there expectantly. "Hello, I'm Nathan. Do you think you could come out and play?" Looking down at my sock feet he suggested, "You might want to put shoes on." Without waiting for a response, he darted off around the corner of the house, leaving me no choice but to hop after him, tying my shoes and smiling in spite of myself.

He got sick the summer we met. When he lost his hair it was still warm outside. We slathered bug spray on in the evenings and he would remind me, "Don't forget my head!" I should confess that I'm not one of "those people" who are enviably graceful and empathetic in the face of illness. If I am unwittingly insensitive, he finds it funnier than he does offensive, and corrects me just as he would my mispronunciation of a paleontology term. We collect rocks, sword fight with sticks, discuss our favorite dinosaurs, and laugh at the silliness of our mothers. We eat cookie dough, jump in leaf piles, throw snowballs, and when we read he curls in the crook of my arm and whispers along with the books he knows by heart.

In February, Nathan was nominated for a Young Heroes award and he asked me to be his date. In the back seat of the family minivan I confessed I was glad his parents were driving, not being a very good driver myself. He commiserated, "Yeah, me neither! My feet don't even reach the pedals. Maybe when I'm five though." When he stoically shook the hand of a four star general after receiving a medal for his continuing courage in the face of seemingly insurmountable illness, I was proud to know him.

On the ride home, we shivered under my coat until the car warmed up debating whose hands and nose were colder. He asked, "Jenna, did you know you're my best friend?" When I said "Nathan, you're mine too," I meant it. As we pulled into my driveway he gave me a carnation, and his little lips collided with my cheek in an exaggerated kissing sound. Stamping my feet in the entryway I watched the van pull away and I thought about the unpredictable nature of love. It is real and unbelievably resilient, it is humorous and also heartbreaking, and for me, it arrived on my front porch peering persistently through my window in the form of a four year old named Nathan.

The stories continue forever. These were just some of the blessings we saw through the people around us.

Families

You meet many amazing families on your journey. You find other families going through the same things that you are dealing with. Some are fighting the same disease, some are fighting another. We found we would be in the hospital in cycles with these families. Sharing this time with them made it manageable. We would share whatever information we had, whether it was funny stories about our children and the hospital staff, or insights on scans and treatments, or just listening to the hard day. Nothing gave us more joy than seeing one of our favorite families finish treatment and go off to have their normal lives back. It never made us sad when we did not see them anymore; they had won their fight and deserved their freedom.

We did notice over time that families dealt with this time differently. We met families who had completed an enormous amount of treatment research and wanted to share all of it with us right now. We met other families that could just sit down and have a normal parent talk. We would discuss the kids' favorite foods, where they would go to school, how they tortured their siblings, and how different chemotherapies would affect them and how to combat it. We met other families that were truly showing God's grace at all times. We would discuss how God was in this journey, but not really causing it. How He could be seen in those little areas, in the details. The most consistent thing about the other families is that each and every one of them wanted to help in some way. Whether it was telling us about treatments or telling us how to survive them, all families wanted the other person's journey to be easier if possible. These talks are the premise for this book.

The best example I have of this is from Nathan himself. Here is how he helped a little girl going through a tough treatment.

Journal entry - *"A few months ago as Nathan was preparing to go through radiation treatment. There was plenty of discussion about whether or not Nathan could do it without anesthesia since he was only four years old. We even tried a full body CT scan to see if he could handle sitting still so long. After plenty of turns and twists, with the help of his doctors and the radiation staff Nathan was able to have two radiation treatments a day for ten days without any anesthesia. It was a true feat for a little boy. The staff, doctors, and we parents were truly amazed at his toughness.*

This past Saturday I was talking with one of the parents I have gotten to know here at the Ronald McDonald House. They have a daughter Nathan's age going through radiation treatment on her head each day for six weeks. Her Dad was telling me that she had just finished her second week and how tough it was. Every day she would have to go in for her "radiation sensitizer" medicine. Then she would wait for two hours before they could go get her radiation "pictures". Then around 3:00 pm she would get knocked out and get her pictures taken. Then she would have to recover from the anesthesia. She would have to do all of this without being able to eat anything. Her Dad was telling me how tough it was for her to not be able to eat at all until dinner time. It was not going well. Her radiation treatments were ten minutes long.

I then relayed Nathan's radiation story. I explained that we had to find "the catch". Whatever it was that would get him to lie still twice a day for treatment with a mask on his face and his head bolted to the table. For Nathan it was stuffed cats. Who knew what it would be for them. I mentioned that the only reason it worked for us was that Nathan's doctors and the radiation staff were on board and really made it happen. When Nathan heard we were discussing something he had done, he interjected what he remembered directly to this little girl. He let her know that it wasn't that bad, especially for a stuffed cat.

These very nice people went in the next day and talked to the doctors. The doctors agreed to try. Then they talked to the radiation staff. And they agreed to try. Then it was her turn. She lay on that table perfectly still for ten minutes and even took a short nap. "If Nathan can do it, so can I". We ran into the family that night after dinner. The smiles were contagious. Her "catch" was planning what she was going to eat every day for breakfast. They are already planning pancakes for tomorrow. The next six weeks have just taken on a much brighter view."

Other Amazing People

We have been blessed with the outpouring of love we have received. Childhood cancer is never a blessing but the people who have touched our lives during this time truly are. Here are some of their stories.

Mother's Day was the day before MIBG therapy. We found ourselves watching the Chicago Cubs play the Philadelphia Phillies. Nathan was not a big baseball fan at the time, he was only four. Therefore, he spent the first inning or so wooing the three wonderful women behind us. I'm not sure they saw much of the game. Nathan had his charm flowing and knew the ladies life stories by the end of the second inning. The four of them spent the whole game talking and playing. These women completely ignored that bald head and the reason for our visit. We found out during the day that they had spent their morning walking the Walk for a Cure. They continued to follow Nathan's story on his Caringbridge site and occasionally sent him notes. It was a very wonderful way to spend Mother's Day and escape from our new reality.

Scott's coworkers wanted to have a "small" party for Nathan just to show their support and visit before Nathan started his Bone Marrow Transplant and to give him "a" gift. To our surprise about thirty people showed up to give him about ten gifts. While there, Nathan was very shy until they handed him a huge wrapped present and asked him to open it. The present was a T-REX Mountain. Nathan became very animated and wanted it to be opened and assembled, *"Now please"*. So, five Air Force engineers that work with Scott opened it and assembled it. Nathan was charming and polite as he said, *"Let me show you where that piece goes"*. They also gave me a Shield of Faith pendant and a dinner out at the Cheesecake Factory. After the mountain was assembled THEY said thank you to us and went back to work.

One day, through the Ronald McDonald House, we were invited by Karri Walsh to the AVP volleyball finals between May/Walsh and Youngs/Branagh at the AVP open in Mason, Ohio. We ventured out into the sun and heat to see the spectacle. Unfortunately, we got there later than we probably should have and the place was packed. The kids had their post BMT green masks on since we were in a crowded area so they looked very conspicuous. We took a lap around the stadium and could not find a single seat for anyone, not even the kids. Not a single person moved over to make room or even look at us. We were on our second lap around and a gentle hand touched my friend's shoulder. She asked, *"What kind of cancer does your son have?"* This mom told us that she just lost her daughter to neuroblastoma and wanted us to take their seats. She would not take no for an answer and guided us over to her seats. Her family and their friends stood at the bottom of the stairs while we got to sit in their place. The match was amazing (May and Walsh lost and ended their winning streak). Through the match, my friend continued to talk with them; it was too tough for me since I cried the whole way to the chairs. We found out later that Nathan and I had met their daughter at the Ronald McDonald house. She and Nathan had played together on many evenings while there.

Your Spouse

Scott and I had been married for 14 years when Nathan was diagnosed with cancer. We had just taken our biggest and best vacation a month before it all began. We thought we were on pretty firm ground as a couple to handle his disease. We had our family and friends to help, we had our church and bible study groups to support us, and we had this amazing medical staff to get us through it. And yet, the question I'm asked the most frequently about this journey, is how did Scott and I stay together through it all. This is a tough journey on anyone. There are soul wrenching days where you feel you child is not going to make it. There are harder days when you just do not want to go to the hospital to care for your child because it is just too hard. I don't think it is even possible to explain in words what a person goes through while watching their child being sick with cancer and going through such difficult treatments that may or may not cure them of this disease.

After the initial diagnosis, Scott and I clung to each other. He was my confidant; he was the only other person that understood what I was going through. He was going through it too. He was there every day, every moment, through everything. We had our talks in great depth about what to do and who should do it. We worked a rotating schedule with the kids where we would alternate nights so we would each get to see Kate. We didn't need to choose the treatment for months, so we were able just to support each other and work out whatever issues we had making day to day life somewhat normal. We had our journal to communicate and let each other know what we were feeling. We got into this autopilot mode of taking care of Nathan and not completely ignoring Kate. We were even able to, on occasion, get someone else to watch the kids while we went to dinner and just chatted with each other. This is not a mode that can be sustained for years, but it worked for us for months. We really only saw each other an hour or so a day.

When we did have the opportunity to be together, whether at the hospital or elsewhere, we tried to reconnect as a couple and not let our circumstances completely get in the way. Sometimes this would be having a cup of coffee in the cafeteria while the kids were being cared for. Sometimes it was more playful. Sometimes, the boys (Nathan and Scott) would hide from me. When I got in range, both of them would jump out and pelt me with Nerf darts and laugh. Usually we would sit quietly while Nathan slept and watch him while just being together. We were best friends. Anytime we were able to do something that was not cancer related rejuvenated us as a couple.

Eventually the stress took its toll. Nathan's treatments were not working as they should. Decisions had to be made by us that were potentially life threatening to Nathan. We were not sure what to do. We did not know how to release this helplessness and anger, so we took it out on each other. We yelled at each other out of pain for our child. We had screaming matches about which treatment options we should pick. One of them came after finishing a phone call with Nathan's doctor. I wanted to talk to Scott more about the treatment and just kept pestering him. In the end, we were yelling at each other not about anything specific but just because our plight looked so very hopeless.

After three years or so of harming our relationship and hurting each other, we did one thing right to mend it and stopped it from being on a free fall to disaster. During a bible study exercise of finding something in our lives we could work on to improve, we chose to finally work on our marriage. It was time to stop taking from the relationship; now it was time to add to the relationship daily. Sometimes it was something small like an intentional and loving kiss on the cheek, *"This is your one nice thing today. We are REALLY busy"*. Sometimes it was bringing home our favorite dessert after a night of volleyball, feeding each other while resting on the couch. It didn't matter really what it was, what mattered is that we were intentionally doing something to show the other one how much we loved them and they knew it. We continue to try to do this still today, but we don't always point them out. It sounds pretty simple, to *intentionally do one explicitly nice thing for your spouse daily*, but it sure does help.

Taking Care of Your Other Children

It can be very easy to get caught up in caring for your sick child and not give your other children the attention they need and deserve. Scott and I would take turns at the hospital with Nathan, which means we were also able to take turns with Kate at home. She was only one year old when Nathan was diagnosed. She does not remember a time when her brother was not sick. I'm not sure how well we did, but I do know that I almost forgot about Nathan's cancer when hanging out alone with Kate. She was so in need of our love and attention. She was so very young and full of life. She wanted and needed her folks to be with her.

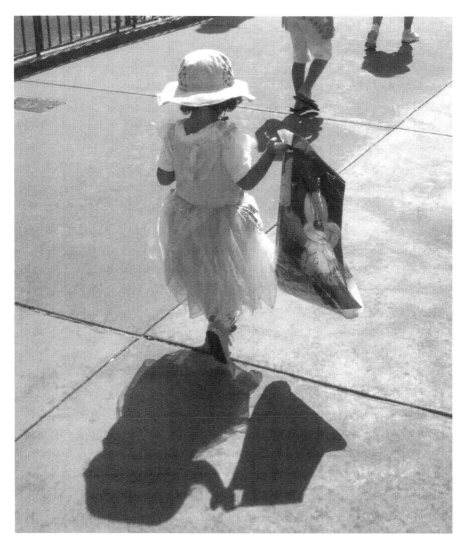

Figure 19 Kate at Disney

This is one area each family needs to figure out for themselves. Every child has different needs and desires. Tough choices have to be made and they are different for everyone. We met families that brought their other young children to the hospital and the whole family was there every day. Some families completely left out the other children to not expose them to what was going on in the hospital. We tried to make Kate's life as "normal" as we could. In every instance, there is some impact on the healthy child or children. We took the philosophy that we would do what we could now and pay the consequence later. We knew some time we would need to address the impact Nathan's disease had on Kate. Now, many years later we are doing this. Kate does have issues, as would be expected.

Journal entry: *"On the other side, Katie is my bright shiny spot. She continues to try all of our patience with the lack of hers. She is constantly making us laugh and grunt in frustration. She still chooses not to really speak, but her understanding of us is HUGE and her sign language vocabulary is growing. It is fun watching her say Help Please without any prompting. She is a doll."*

Kate would find very creative ways to get our attention, or just be a kid, whichever is your perspective. One very memorable event happened at her school with a small bead.

Journal entry: *"I get the call from school… 'Kate has shoved a bead up her nose. It is pretty far up there and we cannot get it out. Please come and see what you can do.' Where the bead came from is still up for debate. They don't have small beads in the little kid's room. Anyway, when I got there the bead was not visible. Kate had shoved it all the way into her sinuses, or so we thought. With nothing to be done at that moment I left Kate at school, she was unwilling to leave, went home to contact her doctors and see what they wanted to do. Kate had found the perfect way to make cancer go away for a few hours. Nathan's care was put on hold while we fished the bead out of Kate's head. Yes, I do still have the report with the bead stuck to it.*

Sometime in the afternoon, she sneezed the bead out of her nose. We did not find this out until after spending time at the doctors where they poked and prodded her face. No one at the school actually saw the bead come out of Kate's head but they did find one on the floor in a corner. They taped it to the incident report and gave it to me.

On the bright side, while at the doctors, we found out that Kate's ear infection is healing nicely."

Even though we kept Kate out of the hospital as much as possible, there are ways to help children visit with each other without visiting the hospital. Children's hospitals usually have many resources available to keep their children happy. Many hospitals have laptop computers the kids can use or have access to a Wi-Fi connection for their own computer. While away from home Nathan would keep in touch with Kate, whichever parent was not at the hospital, and any friends that were around, using a webcam. Whether at a close hospital or further away in another state, he would get up and chat and dance and talk with whomever would chat back.

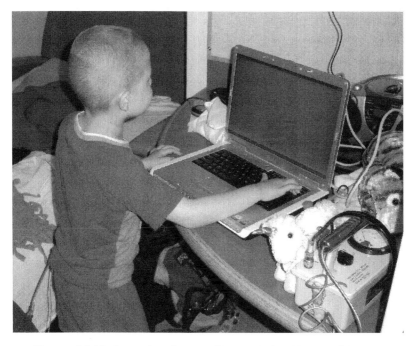

Figure 20 Nathan chatting on line with family and friends.

Primary and Alternate Care Givers

It is unrealistic to think that one adult can adequately care for a child with cancer. It is possible, but very difficult. There needs to be a team.

Identify alternate care givers that will be able to take your child to the doctors when necessary. Find some people, friends, family, neighbors, whomever, who are willing and able to care for your child. Have them identified with the medical staff. Get them trained as needed and to yours and their comfort level. Most people you ask to help or let into your world will be up for the challenge and consider it an honor to be able to help. It is only fair to these folks to have them involved early so they know the routines, are familiar with the doctors and hospital staff, and can be somewhat prepared. It is always tough to leave your sick child at the hospital, but sometimes it just has to happen and a trained friend can make this a lot easier.

My family was very fortunate in this area. The Air Force gave Scott as much time off work as he needed to care for his family. Scott was up for a deployment during BMT. Another Air Force officer volunteered so that Scott could be around to care for us. Scott was able to participate fully in Nathan's care each and every step along the way. We also had Scott's mother full time to help. She quit her job and moved to be with us through the worst part of treatment. I have heard of many families where grandparents take any other children home with them so that parents can concentrate on caring for their sick child during BMT and other times during treatment.

Even with all this support, after a year or so it was not surprising that I started to come down with interesting illnesses. I developed abdominal cysts that would burst. It is not possible to take your child to chemotherapy when you are curled up in a bed in the ER on six doses of morphine; you need someone to help. There may be other times when your sisters require you to run away to Atlantic City kicking and screaming because they know how much you love the ocean and they know you need to see it. The unexpected will happen. It is always better to have a plan than to make it up as you go and to have people who know what to do when you call.

We were also fortunate to have friends to help us. One very dear family took care of Kate frequently. Sometimes Scott and I could not get to her day care to pick her up before it closed. They would. They did not take Nathan to the hospital but the sure took care of Kate and me when necessary. Our journey would have been so much more difficult without them.

Accepting Help

If you are like us, asking for and receiving help from others can be a very difficult and uncomfortable emotional task. We were the people that would jump into any project and do whatever it takes to get the job done. It was really not our way to be on the receiving end. We are very glad we got over this; we cannot imagine trying to accomplish this alone. As I mentioned above, when Nathan was first sent to the hospital, Scott was out of town and Kate was just a little baby. Our need for help started right there with a call out of the blue to a friend to watch Kate, not just for a few hours but for the entire night. Our friends were very open and gave their home to Kate while I spent the night in the hospital with Nathan. Then there were the countless meals from all the friends. The spouses club from the Air Force would come and take care of things for us, our Bible study groups would take their turns, and then the neighborhood would do our yard and watch the kids when we were home so we could sleep. Not only did it really help us out, but I was told by many of our friends they were so grateful that there was something they could do that would ease our burden just a little bit.

We did find when people asked us what they can do, we really didn't know. It wasn't that we were trying to be strong, we just never had an answer to the generic question *"Is there anything we can do for you?"* We were living one moment at a time and really did not think ahead as to what needed to be done longer term. It was always easier when a friend would ask us if they could do something specific for us like rake leaves, bring a meal, check the mail, water the yard, make a small grocery run, or simply sit in the house for parent rest time. Since our journey was long and drawn out, our friends were great at figuring this out and finding something to do. The funniest time was a couple years into treatment. I needed to have a small surgical procedure that would keep me down for about six weeks recovering. Scott was deployed for six months when my surgery date came up. My wonderful volleyball

Bible study friends knew I had become tired of accepting help all the time, so they scheduled a yard clean up right after my surgery so that I could not say no. This group was one of the bright spots for help and love and prayer. They told me they felt privileged that we let them walk this walk with us.

Remember this: when people ask to help, let them, and cherish the time with them as best as you can. For the people offering help, remember to offer something specific. It is easier for the recipient to say yes or no than it is to come up with an idea of help without feeling like they are taking advantage of you.

Crazy Things Can Happen

Most parents can be very protective during such a difficult trial. We tried to shield our children from any and all harm. Granted we were going to have to let our child go through cancer treatment that was going to make him very sick and have all sorts of consequences, but we felt we could keep the rest of life's dangers away from both of them. We were wrong. There is no way you can predict all the hazards and weird things your child will face and prevent them from happening. The best thing we found to do was to have a plan in place and follow it when crazy things did happen. Here are a couple examples.

Nathan's Broviac Catheter vs. the Slide

Nathan was one week away from going for MIBG therapy followed by BMT. We had kept him healthy, his numbers had recovered, and he was as ready to start treatment as he could be. One evening, while we were in our sun room Nathan was on the swing set playing. When we heard him scream Scott was at his side immediately. Nathan had gotten his Broviac catheter caught in the slide as he went down the slide and was hanging by it when we got to him. (Broviac catheter has the tubes dangling outside the body.) The worst went through my head. When Scott picked him up and turned him over I expected to see blood and lots of it. I expected to see his line out of his chest. Scott picked him up, I got his line unstuck and we carried him inside. No blood, just one terrified little boy, parents and grandmother. We immediately called the oncologist and told him our story. We ended up in the ED that evening just to make sure the end of the line was still properly in place. It was. Nathan was fine. A very small part of the line was now exposed which had not been before. It was not what they call the cuff, just a fatter part of the line. We talked about replacing his line, we had it x-rayed, and we had IV therapist look at it. In the end, everyone agreed it was fine and we moved on. So, how did we prevent this from happening again? Nathan wore bib overalls every day after the slide incident until his Broviac catheter was removed. We were not taking any more chances. When it was removed, months later, to be replaced with a port catheter, we found the Broviac had been securely in place even after the slide.

Your Health and Stress

It is difficult to imagine the stress your body is put through during the care for your child. You miss hours and days of sleep, you worry, you pace the floor, you do things that you thought were not possible. When Kate was born, I was one month shy of 40 years old. I thought that I was tired caring for such a young baby. Later, I realized those were the days when I got the most sleep in years. This stress you are under might impact your own health. You cannot predict how the stress will manifest itself. Try to take care of yourself as much as possible, because if you do get sick, you cannot bring those germs to the hospital with you.

One thing I learned was if a doctor asks you if you are sick, you should probably listen. Once while sitting in an appointment with Nathan, his doctor asked me if I was sick. I, of course, just pushed the comment off and said it was allergies or something else not worth addressing. A couple days later I was diagnosed with pneumonia in my right lung. I was sick for many weeks and had to slow down and rest more and not try to do everything myself.

Another time Nathan and I arrived at the Oncology Clinic to have Nathan's chemotherapy. When I walked in the staff asked me, "*What bus hit you?*" Once again, I said I was fine just a bit tired and would be fine, don't worry about me. Later that week, a cyst that had been bleeding internally the whole week burst. That was a surreal moment in my life. I was lying in the Emergency Room while they figured out what was wrong with me and causing all the pain. Scott had to leave me there since he had to take Nathan to the hospital for chemotherapy. Only in the world of childhood cancer is that level of pain a lot less important than your child's care.

Programs for Kids

I do not try to imagine this journey through Nathan's perspective. I just assume it is horrible and assume that anything we can do to cheer him up is a good thing. In the hospital or community, there are many programs for children in many different forms. Use them; they are there to make your child feel better, even if only for a moment. Nathan's hospital had programs like "Caps for Kids," where there are baseball caps signed by different sport stars or other celebrities. Nathan chose a hat from Derek Lee, his favorite baseball player.

Some hospitals have an Emily's Beads of Courage or Beads of Courage program where a child gets a certain type of bead for each of the things that happen to them during treatment. He would get a bead for each "poke", a bead for each dose of chemotherapy, a bead for radiation therapy, and so on. Nathan loved to collect these beads and compare them to his friends' beads. Emily Beads of Courage also had events such as going to a local baseball game as a group and having a barbeque. The kids get baseball hats, food, and games.

Some hospitals have summer camp for Hematology/Oncology patients. The camp has doctors and nurses there on site 24 hours a day, 7 days a week, to administer medications and care for any ailment. No parents attend. The kids get to be kids for a whole week with other kids that are just like them.

Another program we have been involved with is Waves of Hope. Local boat owners plan a boat outing. They pick up kids and their siblings and parents at the marina. They show them a day of boating, BBQ and beach fun.

These are just a few we have been privileged to work with. Organizations are out there that LOVE to spoil kids. Check with your hospital staff to see what is available in your area and how they can participate. Check with your child's doctor to make sure they are well enough to participate, but, in general, any distraction during treatment is a good thing.

Hospital Humor

Granted, there is very little to laugh about chemotherapy, ED visits, side effects, treatment options, and so on. However, sometimes, something so silly comes along you just need to allow yourself to see it for the humor it contains. If you can take the cancer out of some events, they can appear quite humorous. Nathan and Kate supplied us with many stories. Here are a couple that stand out.

Flu Shots

Nathan is a tough kid. He goes through therapy without complaint. He has blood drawn and smiles and laughs with the nurses as they care for him. He takes his chemotherapy, feels horrible and asks if I'm feeling all right; *"What is wrong mom?"* During his bone marrow transplant, he was lying in bed curled up in a ball clearly in pain. When I asked him if he was in pain and could I help him, he said *"No mom, I'm fine."* This kid is tough. We did find one kink in his armor, flu shots! When Nathan's immune system was strong enough, he could get his flu shot in the fall. The first time I remember so clearly. We put cream on his arm to numb the area. When the nurse came in to give him the shot, Nathan started to scream as loudly as he could. It was so bad almost the entire staff came to check on him (many had never heard him cry). When we decided that he was not going to be calmed down, we agreed to just give him the shot. I had him in a body hug to keep his arms and legs from thrashing. The nurse gave him his shot and he continued to scream. Another five minutes went by before he would even talk. He could finally catch his breath and screamed, "Is it done yet?!" So, my tough little boy was screaming for ten minutes and never even felt the shot. It is the same thing every year.

Kate had the exact opposite opinion of flu shots. Kate had a very warped perspective of doctors and what visiting the hospital was like. Since Scott and I had spent many hours in the hospital with Nathan, she felt it must be fun, all that time with mom or dad. We understood that it was not fun and was usually very boring. It was very difficult to convince Kate of this. Whenever possible we would allow Kate to join us at the hospital and even get her vitals taken. She did not like any of it, but she still thought it was supposed to be fun. It was especially exciting for her when it was flu shot time.

Journal entry - *"I don't know how many of you have chatted with Kate about the doctors, but she thinks going to the doctor is the greatest thing ever. Since Nathan and I go all the time alone, it must be so very fun. The mole on her right leg has been bandaged almost every night so she had something medical to take care of too. Well, yesterday was her time to go to the doctor to get her flu shot. She was giggling and chanting at school all day. "I'm going to the doctor, I'm getting a shot" (put to song). She was so excited. The time finally came. We were at the hospital from 2:00pm to 7:00pm. She did very well considering it was her first long day at the hospital. She did not like the blood pressure cuff. She DID NOT like her shot. And in general she wanted to go home about three hours before we left. But she did great for the shot. She sat there and took the shot silently. Then they pulled the shot out and threw the needle away. Then it set in that it HURT!!! She screamed but only for a minute. Then she continued with the task of annoying her brother."*

Daily Accomplishments

Some days it is a good idea to have low expectations of things you want to accomplish. Many days it is just not going to happen. Instead of spending that day being frustrated because you are accomplishing nothing, set you goals lower and delight in accomplishing those.

Journal entry – *"We are still home. Nathan and I are both in weird moods after being in the hospital for most of a week. We went out and got some milk as our accomplishment for the day."*

Journal entry – *"Well, we made it one day without going to a hospital."*

Use Medical Supplies for Fun

After months and months of being worried nonstop and being intimidated with all the medical supplies and equipment, you do eventually start incorporating things into your now normal daily routine. Nathan and Scott were very good at turning syringes into all kinds of toys, water guns, noise makers, and - one time - a rocket.

Journal entry– "HOW MY BOY INVENTS A ROCKET!

This evening after Scott finished giving Nathan his medicine, Scott was showing Nathan how you can pull back on the capped syringe and it will make a very loud noise as the plunger goes slamming back to fill the vacuum. Nathan then says, "But, Daddy, if you let go of the syringe as it goes back I bet it will fly across the room". And you know what? It does. It even flies across the living room and kitchen. And still makes the very loud noise as it goes. This can entertain a four year old and a 39 year old for a VERY long time as they try to hit Mommy while she does the dishes. Their aim got VERY good."

Take Them to a Fancy Dinner

Mommy: "Hey, Nathan, what do you want to do for your birthday? Do you want to get nuggets to take back to the house or do you want to go out for a fancy dinner?"

Nathan: "How about a fancy dinner, Mom."

Mommy: "Ooo, that sounds fun. Where do you want to go for a fancy dinner?"

Nathan: "McDonalds!"

Laugh at Their Jokes.

Mommy: Nathan what is for dessert?

Nathan: You know, Mom, it is that little sweet thing you have after having good stuff for dinner.

Sometimes You Just Let Them Win

After spending so much time in the hospital, the kids become accustomed to it. They start to figure out how to do things for themselves, regardless of the "reasonable" explanation you give them for why they cannot do something. Nathan was exceptional at this. While he was in the radiation phase of his treatment he wanted a bath. "*Sorry, Nathan, you cannot have a bath, you cannot wash off the radiation marks. They need them to line things up.*" He gave me some time before coming back at me again asking for a bath. "*I'm Sorry Nathan, but there are no bathtubs here at this hospital.*" Not to be deterred, he now had a place he could argue. Now he had a plan. "*Mom, if we filled a pink bucket with water, I could take a bath in it. My radiation marks will stay out of the water. And Mom, if we put it in the bathroom, there is a drain there and we won't make a mess. And, Mom, if we use a second bucket, I can wash my feet. And, Mom, if we have a third bucket I can fill a cup with water and pour it over me.*" And here you have Nathan taking that bath in his three pink buckets.

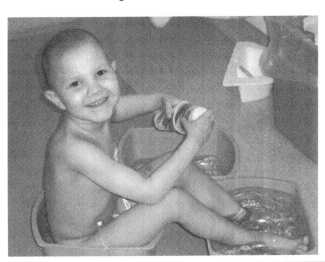

NOTES

NOTES

NOTES

NOTES

CHAPTER 6. TYPES OF MEDICINES

Phased Studies

Phased Studies, sometime called Clinical Trials, are part of the process through which a drug or medicine completes to be approved by the Food and Drug Administration (FDA). Once approved it can be prescribed by doctors for patients. A drug cannot be given to children until it is proven to be safe. Each type of phased studies has a specific objective to prove the drug, when given correctly, will not harm your child and later to prove it effective in treating the disease. They generally come in three parts:

Phase I – safety
Phase II – effectiveness
Phase III – is it better than what is used

Once complete it becomes a Standard of Care that can be prescribed by a doctor without having to be on a study to get it.

You may ask, *"Why would I want to put my child on a study?"* The reason is that many of the treatments available for your child can only be accessed through a study. Neuroblastoma treatment is still evolving. Therefore, somewhere in the battle with neuroblastoma the best, most promising treatment may only be available through a study. In the end, trials are great if they work, trials are horrible if they fail and no one knows which is which before they are run. The best way to decide whether or not to put your child on a phased study is to talk to your medical staff. Get informed. Find out the objectives and how they impact your child. Find out everything you can about the trial and study drug. This is one area in the treatment journey during which there are never too many questions.

There are at least three organizations that specialize in studies for children with neuroblastoma. Their name or acronym is found with a number and title of a study. When researching treatment options and studies, each of these organizations may present different options.

The contact information for each organization can be found in Chapter 9 of this book.

- Children's Oncology Group (COG). This organization works with the NCI to fund pediatrics trials for many types of childhood cancer.
- Neuroblastoma Medulloblastoma Translational Research Consortium (NMTRC). The NMTRC is a group of universities and children's hospitals to research treatments for specifically neuroblastoma and medulloblastoma.
- New Approaches to Neuroblastoma Therapy (NANT). It is a different group of universities and children's hospitals focused on finding treatments for neuroblastoma.

Phase I

The main objective of a Phase I study is to determine the safety of a new drug or treatment. It is designed to show how much of the drug can be given safely to a child without unacceptable toxicities or adverse side effects. This is usually done in stages of dose escalation of the drug or drug combination. Dose escalation is when doses start small and escalate on a timeline to a point where it has reached the maximum dose, or it is proven unsafe. The first dosages are usually relatively low and safe. Once the doctors are comfortable with this dose level, the next level is started as defined in the protocol and so on. When there are "dose limiting toxicities", a Phase I study is stopped. Dose limiting toxicity is when the side effects are severe enough to harm the child. In general, the acceptable dose for this drug is then set to the previous dose in the protocol. This will be the starting point for the Phase II part of the study. Let me clarify, Phase I studies do not explicitly deal with effectiveness of the treatment drug.

A big problem with Phase I studies is the insurance coverage. Many insurance companies do not cover Phase I trials. They are considered highly experimental. Drug companies usually cover the cost of the drug itself; however, the additional care, scans, tests, etc. may not be covered by insurance if part of a phase I study. Check with your insurance company to make sure you understand their policies. Coverage can be negotiated if necessary. For example: we worked with a group called the Patient Advocate Foundation to get coverage for those things that would have also been covered on a Phase II trial. (http://www.patientadvocate.org/). Work with anyone who can help you through the tremendous amount of information regarding which trials are right for you and how to get insurance coverage when needed.

Nathan was on one Phase I study for antibody therapy. The study was a modification to the standard antibody treatment which targeted boney lesions. The phase I part of the treatment was the addition of a new drug that Nathan called his "super glue" medicine. The point of the drug was to help the antibodies stick to the cancer cells long enough to let the body kill them. We were able to convince the insurance company to cover the Phase II part of the study and we would cover the experimental part.

Phase II

The main objective of a Phase II study is to determine the effectiveness of a drug while continuing to evaluate the safety of the dose levels determined in the Phase I trial. Phase II studies are usually available to more patients through more hospitals than a Phase I study.

In a Phase II study, all aspects are generally planned out to prove the drug works and determine the side effects. Scans are scheduled; tests must be conducted at specific times and so on. There are nuances to a Phase II trial. For example, you are not allowed to add any other types of treatment while on a Phase II study, mainly because if you are on another treatment drug it is impossible to determine which drug is doing what to your child. There may be a time at which you have to decide if it is best for your child to stay on study and deal with treatment as detailed, or remove them from the study because something else is better for your child. Do not make these decisions rashly, once you leave a study it is generally not possible to get back on it. Once again, discuss these issues with the doctors and staff in order to make the best choice for your child.

Nathan has been on a couple Phase II trials. We did take him off one of the trials early. His MIBG and BMT therapy was a Phase II study. It was clear from the first set of scans after his BMT that he had completely failed the study. He was supposed to be clear of disease and ready for radiation treatment. However, he still had disease scattered throughout his entire body. The study stated specific things that Nathan needed to do post BMT but all were related to healing and recovery. Unfortunately for us, he was not in the healing and recovery phase of Nathan's care and we needed to come up with a new plan. There were many things Nathan had to complete to leave the study, just like there were many to get onto the study. His doctor and the hospital staff were exceptional, being considerate of our plight rather than making the study the important part. They did what was needed to be done by the study guidelines and completed the paperwork, mostly without us knowing it. There were a few occasions when we needed a new study, blood test, scan or whatever to remove Nathan from the trial, but they were done in conjunction of things he needed to complete for his follow on care.

The other phase II study was for a drug called ABT-751. It is an immunotherapy drug designed to prevent progression. More about ABT-751 later.

Phase III

The main objective of a Phase III study is to compare the current drug or treatment plan to the "standard of care" to see if it works better. These are considered blind studies where you are picked randomly for one of the two different arms of treatment. One arm is the current standard of care while the other arm is the new treatment protocol. These trials continue until the defined completion date, or when it is shown that the new treatment is statistically better or worse than the old study.

Nathan was not on any phase III studies during his treatment.

Enrollment Requirements

All studies are not open to all patients. Generally, the group studying the drug has a very specific group of patients in mind that their drug will help the most, or the drug will be easiest to prove with, or some other criteria for running the trial. Many trials are for patients with chemotherapy resistant disease also called refractory disease, or have progression. Your medical team will be able to help navigate through the trial options and enrollment criteria and how they apply to your child.

We wanted Nathan on a Phase II study and were going through the normal process of enrolling him. We signed the consent forms to start evaluating Nathan for treatment. Since his disease was still scattered throughout his bones, we expected no problems. However, one of the requirements for enrollment was proof of active disease. This seemed straight forward enough except his bone marrow biopsy test results had been inconclusive as to whether or not it was positive or negative, right side or left side, etc. It was an interesting change of mindset to actually hope for his bone marrow results to be positive so that he could start on the trial sooner rather than later. In this case, Nathan's bone marrow biopsy originally came back negative. The biopsy involves taking a 1 cm deep core out of his bone. They then take micron slices from this core and look for neuroblastoma cells. The first couple micron thick slices did not have any cells. Nathan's doctor spoke with the pathologist and asked them to take a few more slices to see if he can find any neuroblastoma cells. Later that day, they did find some cells in his additional slices. With these few cells, Nathan was able to start his Phase II study without further testing.

FDA Approved Drugs

Once a drug has been put through all three drug trial phases, it can be prescribed by a doctor as part of your child's care, and your child would no longer be required to be on a trial to get it. There are many treatments available that are no longer part of a phased trial. After Nathan completed his frontline therapy, he still had significant disease throughout his body. The doctor chose other chemotherapy drugs, available without a trial, to treat Nathan, while we figured out what to do next. These chemotherapy drugs had already been approved by the FDA (Food and Drug Administration) and were available to the doctors to treat Nathan.

Other Non-cancer Drug used to Fight Cancer

There are many stories out there about medicines that fight cancer but are not chemotherapies. If any of them sound like a good idea to try on your child, ask your doctor before using them. The doctors will be able to determine if the medicines are safe and give you their educated opinions on whether they feel the drug will help. They may have very promising potential to help, but they may also inhibit your child's current treatment and actually reduce the effectiveness of them. In the worst case, they could negatively interact with the chemotherapy and harm your child.

Supplements

There are many supplements on the market that claim to work on different forms of cancer. Please do not hide any of these supplements you want to give your child from their medical staff. There may be a known interaction with the drugs your child is being given or other factors that the doctors need to know while under their care. As with the non-cancer drugs above, there may be potential for helping, but you may also inadvertently hurt your child's treatment.

Researching Treatments

As you proceed through different stages of treatment you find many parents with kids in varying stages of therapy. Some will be just staring with frontline therapy, others will be almost completed and still others will be dealing with a relapse. You will find very enthusiastic parents that have been at this for years and have researched everything available. Try not to be intimidated by this and do not feel you need to do the same, especially at the early stages of treatment. Take care of your child, yourself, and your family. Rely on the doctors and staff you have to help you until you are ready to venture into the area of online research. The amount of data out there is very overwhelming. It is even more difficult to find the specific information you want that applies to your case.

Do your research, read the papers, talk to parents and doctors involved in the research, but in the end you need to discuss things with your doctor who can then be your advocate in getting them implemented.

There is no magic cure to cancer. As I have mentioned above, the best chance for a cure is frontline therapy. Therefore, spend your time and energy on these treatments until they are no longer working. Each treatment will hopefully take you one step closer to having "no evidence of disease" (NED).

When Treatment Does Not go as Planned

When treatment starts with frontline therapy, most decisions are made for you. There is a standard of care to follow that is considered the best treatment plan for your child at this time. However, there may come a day when your child's neuroblastoma is not responding acceptably to that treatment and you need to find other treatment options. There are many other options out there. It is important to talk with your doctors to find out what to do next. Be informed. Learn what you can about each option and do not be afraid to share your opinion with the doctors. In the end, it is your choice. Here is our story, the long, not straight path through childhood cancer treatment.

Nathan's story

I have mentioned bits and pieces of Nathan's treatment in the sections above. Here I would like to show you his path through treatments and medicines to give a better timeline and overview of what he has gone through.

Nathan was diagnosed on August 8, 2006. The first few months proceeded as planned. The surgeon was able to completely remove his primary tumor and put in his intravenous catheter. Chemotherapy started. He had two rounds of chemotherapy followed by his stem cells harvest. Four more rounds of varying chemotherapies as defined in the protocol. Treatments and side effects were just as expected. All went as expected until we started preparing for BMT. We learned that Nathan did not have a lot of success on frontline therapy. The treatments did not work quite the way they were supposed to. Each treatment only worked to a certain degree, and, with the help of our medical team, we came up with one alternative and then another.

When frontline therapy was over, Nathan's scans showed disease still riddled throughout his skeleton. His disease load was significantly lower, but still too high to go into bone marrow transplant. The worst possible scenario would be to go through BMT and still have active disease throughout his body. Then he would still have to fight but would have nothing to fight with because his immune system would be very weak. While researching treatments, we came across a different cocktail of chemotherapy which was not part of frontline therapy. He had a few rounds of it while we figured out what to do next. It also reduced his disease load a bit more.

With the help of our two most trusted doctors, we came up with a new plan. There was a Phase II study that would include MIBG therapy just before bone marrow transplant. It would be timed so that both treatments would have Nathan's blood counts going towards zero around the same time. This was a big risk for us. If the MIBG therapy did not reduce the disease load such that BMT could wipe out the remaining disease, we would once again be in the worst possible scenario. However, in our opinion, and our doctors' opinions, this was Nathan's best chance to have a cure.

As with all of Nathan's treatments, it worked a bit, but did not clear his disease. The first set of scans following BMT still showed disease throughout his skeleton and his bone marrow was still positive for disease. He was supposed to do radiation next, but there was too much disease to radiate.

By this point in our journey, we had met and worked with many different doctors. We weighed pros and cons from each of their opinions. In the end, we kept coming back to two doctors. Their opinions and advice tended to work. We worked with them best. We trusted them and weighed their opinions higher than the rest. When at a cross roads like we were post BMT, we would find reasons to put ourselves in contact with these two doctors, in person. When you get that far off the primary treatment path, there are a lot of options out there and no one person knows which treatment is going to work. Each treatment option may or may not work on your child's cancer. Your child's cancer is different than another child's cancer. Each patient is very unique.

With disease throughout Nathan's body and bone marrow after BMT and MIBG therapy, there were no more "big gun" therapies left. We were living out our worst case scenario. We needed a completely new treatment plan. We needed something that was not as caustic as chemotherapy but would hold this disease off. We were presented with a few different options from the doctors. None of them sounded promising, and all of them sounded like we were just giving up, except one. The one we chose was the most risky. We were going to have Nathan go through another round of high dose chemotherapy and another stem cell rescue. Nathan would also have radiation therapy in specific worrisome areas instead of all the remaining disease since Nathan had too much disease left to radiate it all. We were then going to go to another hospital for a Phase I antibody treatment. The treatment we had chosen was only available in one hospital. The biggest concern was whether Nathan was strong enough to get through the high dose chemotherapy right after finishing BMT. We felt that he could survive this, and it was truly our only option. We believed if we did not do this treatment at this point of time against Nathan's neuroblastoma, we would lose this option. It was take it now or never take it.

We had one big decision left, and that was where to do the high risk chemotherapy and radiation. Do we do it at our home hospital where the doctor completely agrees with the treatment plan? Life would be easier for us and we would get to see Kate, but we would need to travel twice a day 45 minutes away for radiation. Or, do we do it at the BMT hospital where the doctor did not necessarily agree with our treatment option? It would probably be the safest place to have it done, but we would be away from home another month and we were ready to no longer be in that hospital. How to make this decision? Not only that, how do you even proceed to get a treatment plan in place specified by doctors that are states away? What paperwork would we need, and how long would it take to implement it? Who would coordinate all the different types of treatment? Who would be in charge when the doctor dictating the treatment wasn't even in this hospital? Who would deal with insurance?

I arrived at one of Nathan's post BMT meetings to ask some of these questions and tell the doctor that our decision was to do the treatment at our home hospital (not the BMT hospital). We wanted some normalcy and to see Kate. Before I was able to finalize this decision, the doctor told me the answer to all the above questions. I was informed how many documents would need to be done and who would need to sign them. I was told of all the dangers and the coordinating issues. I was told of issues I had not thought about. I now had even more things to resolve than before. Then the doctor handed me all the signed documents I would need for the treatment to be done at the BMT hospital. The plan was already in place and all I had to do was agree to it, so, I did. It was an excellent choice on our part. The very first evening of Nathan's high dose chemotherapy he spiked a 104F fever. He stayed in the hospital for four weeks.

Treatment went according to plan. Nathan had high dose chemotherapy followed by a stem cell rescue. He then had radiation treatments twice a day for ten days. He enjoyed these because he got to take an ambulance to the radiation center two times a day. Once all chemotherapy and radiation was completed, we traveled to yet another hospital for his antibody therapy. He ended up having four rounds of antibody therapy before beginning to have enough negative reactions (toxicities) to the treatment that it had to be stopped.

After six months, this new treatment plan was done. Once again, treatment worked a bit, but did not cure Nathan of cancer. Antibody therapy was states away from home and very tough. We were all exhausted physically and mentally and we still had this horrible disease throughout Nathan's body. It was smaller, but it was still there and Nathan's bone marrow was still positive for neuroblastoma.

We were then back to the doctors, back to asking questions, and back to researching treatments on the Internet. The one thing we did have this time was that Nathan was a bit stronger; he was almost a year past BMT. But it was time to find something other than chemotherapy for him. We had been poisoning him for almost two years and it just was not killing the cancer. We had tried all the proven treatments, and he was not clear of disease. We were now entering the area of experimental medicine. No one knew which therapies would work and which therapies would not work. We were down to the very last options available for Nathan. In the end, we came to two choices. There were two Phase II studies that looked a little more promising than taking Nathan off all treatment completely. We were fortunate enough to meet the lead doctor of one of the studies at a parent neuroblastoma conference. He informed us that in his opinion his study was not far enough along for Nathan. He recommended we try the other Phase II study first, and, when we were done with that, hopefully, his study would be ready for us. So, that is what we did.

Nathan started his Phase II study in August of 2008. The drug was designed to keep Nathan's disease stable. It was not designed to kill the neuroblastoma, just keep it from growing too quickly. We expected Nathan to be able to take this drug for at least eight rounds. At least we hoped for eight rounds. That would give us six months to decide what to do next, not that there were many options left. The next six months went very slowly. Every ache, every pain, every twitch, every complaint from Nathan immediately made us think that he was progressing and our fight was over. However, those eight rounds came and went and Nathan continued to be stable. Then, another eight rounds came and went and still stable. After two years on this treatment, the drug company completed the study. The drug had completely failed. Of the 95 or so children on the drug, it had helped one. Nathan was the only documented case we heard of responding to this drug at all. Not only did it keep Nathan's disease stable, it cleared many tumor beds. We were going to keep him on this drug as long as we could.

Now there was a new problem. We had a drug that worked on Nathan, but the study was ending. The staff at our hospital worked with the drug manufacturer and the FDA to get a compassionate use waiver for Nathan. They effectively created a study for one person, Nathan. He was going to be able to continue on this drug until the company stopped making it. That bought us three more years. It brings us to now. He is still on this drug. We continue to work with the doctors to decide what comes next or when to stop his treatment. He still has MIBG positive disease in his femurs and tibias, but it is very slight.

He continues to fight!

NOTES

NOTES

CHAPTER 7. LATE EFFECTS

Throughout treatment, many of the side effects of the medicines are obvious and short term. The blood counts drop but rise again, fevers come and go, pain is more and less, and so on. There are many other side effects which may not be as obvious and may show up later. These are called late effects or long term side effects. Hearing and vision loss, learning issues, attention span issues, muscle atrophy, radiation damage and the like are considered late effects. These late effects are well documented; they exist and affect the entire family. We have not found as much information on how to handle or treat them as we have about the fact they exist. The following sections are what we have learned over the past few years as Nathan has entered school. These sections are our own personal experiences with late effects and are by no means inclusive.

Hearing Loss

A very common side effect of the intense chemotherapy is hearing loss. Nathan has severe loss at the higher frequencies and down to moderate loss at the lower frequencies. Nathan's hearing was tested less than six months after treatment started. He was placed in a silent room with headphones on. The audiologist talked with him and ran tests using sounds at many different frequencies. For little kids like Nathan, they play games where the child places a toy in a box when the sound is heard. At the six month point, Nathan's hearing had already dropped significantly. It is very disheartening as a mom sitting in the room of his hearing tests, hearing the noise on the other side of the room, through his head phones when he could not hear them with the headphones on.

After discussing his case with the audiologist, we felt the best plan for Nathan was to get him hearing aids to help at the high frequencies. He has good hearing at the lower frequencies and so we want him to use his natural hearing as best he can at those frequencies. The hearing aids work by taking those higher frequencies and shifting them to the lower range where he hears well. Because he does have a lot of hearing left, the ear molds for the hearing aids are open in the center so sounds can filter directly to his ear. As the years go by the hearing aid technology has improved to help him more. Now his hearing aids can connect via blue tooth to some devices, so he hears the sound directly from his hearing aid instead of through the air.

Hearing aids put your child in a special category at school. They are now hearing impaired. This allows your child to receive special care at school. The special needs instructor/teacher/supervisor should be able to tell you the resources available for your child. In Nathan's case, his class has an FM system in the room. The teacher talks into the microphone, and the sound comes out over a loud speaker in the class room. According to Nathan, it helps the whole class. The other students use a microphone when they are reading aloud so Nathan can now hear them, where without the FM system he could not.

Nathan enjoyed picking out hearing aids. He was allowed to pick the color of the hearing aids themselves and the molds that go into his ears. As with most things in this journey, figuring out the hearing aids had their own problems. He didn't like them, they hurt his ears, and he could not get them in right. A little love and perseverance and a lot of bribery for the four year old helped get us through. We met with our audiologist as often as we needed to get Nathan to accept his new help. Initially, we were very careful not to push him too hard to wear them all the time. We felt that over time he would see how much they helped him and would come to use them more and more on his own. Now, years later, Nathan understands how they help him and wears them most of the time without being told to. We have his hearing checked annually around school time and keep track of changes, which has been minor since the chemotherapy has ended.

The last bit of advice I have about hearing is for the parents and family. It can get very aggravating listening to your child say "what" all the time, or having to repeat yourself constantly, or having to wave your hands to get their attention because they have headphones on. Remember, they are not faking the hearing loss. Being a mom, it is even harder; usually the loss is at higher frequencies, a mom's voice level. You need to remember to treat your child like they have hearing loss. The hearing aids help but they do not cure the hearing loss. Please accept that you must treat them differently when it comes to hearing. They may not do well in crowded places or large groups; they just cannot make out what people are saying. They may just go along with whatever is going on around them because they cannot hear any differently and therefore will frequently be in the wrong place. Please be their biggest advocate in their hearing loss, not their biggest critic.

Learning

Nathan has had a lot of learning difficulties since he finished his chemotherapy regime. Before chemotherapy, he was a very quick learner. We could read a book to him once and he would recite it back to us. We told him something about science or the world around him and he would tell us all about it as if it were his idea the next time we talked. He was bright and loved to learn anything. One time when we were at the clinic for chemotherapy, there was a little boy named Thomas going through the same stuff but was a couple years ahead of Nathan in the treatment timeline. He had a tutor to help with school work. Nathan invited himself to be part of this session. The tutor was talking about rhyming words and was asking Thomas which words rhyme. Thomas was having a very tough time grasping this new, and what appeared to be difficult, concept of rhyming. One of the sets of words was "road" and "run". Nathan interrupted, "That is not a rhyme; that is alliteration". The tutor was very proud of my four year old and continued with her lesson. Now that Nathan is finished with chemotherapy and bone marrow transplant, he has a lot of the same learning issues that I saw in Thomas that day. My first bit of advice is to realize these learning issues are real. The kids are not faking it. Be patient; it is more frustrating for them than you. This learning difficulty is commonly called chemo brain or chemo fog. From what Nathan has told me, it is like having a fuzzy brain or feeling like he just woke up and cannot concentrate. The bad news is that it does not completely go away. The good news is there are ways to learn around or through it.

We saw our first indication of Nathan's learning issues when he was starting to read. He would get stuck on "book." He had a great trouble with the "-ook" words. He would spend two minutes trying to sound the word out. Finally, he would be able to grasp this word and move on. The next sentence had the same word and we would go through the same two minute sound out period. We were thinking to ourselves that there is NO WAY he forgot the word in one sentence. We thought he was just being difficult and not wanting to read, when in fact he was having terrible trouble with this and could not get it. This is an area in which great patience is required. You must try to make this fun. You must make it a positive experience. It is not their fault.

Things continued to be bad as he tried to read. He was about to enter first grade. This was a joyous time in our lives. We never expected him to make it to kindergarten, first grade was a dream come true. Now his learning problems were full blown and causing a lot of difficulty at school. We continued to see the same issues at home and still thought he was just being difficult. We decided to talk to the school about having him tested. They asked me what we wanted him tested for. I replied that we wanted to test him for anything they could test him for, anything from IQ to physical therapy. I was interested in finding out where he was mentally and physically. We wanted a direction on where best to spend our time to help him. We were pleasantly surprised that the school said yes and proceeded to test him. (I did learn later that a school is required by law to test a child if the parent asks them to do it.) When we received the tests back, we were very depressed when we found out our little miracle of a boy failed every test. He had short term memory issues. He had attention span issues. He had processing speed issues. He could not hold a pencil right. He could not run across the gym. He failed all but one test, IQ. His IQ was fine. He was smart. Once something was in his brain he could use it. Now we needed to figure out how to get things into that brain.

We started addressing his issues. He was put on an Individual Education Plan (IEP). His teacher was informed of his issues and how to work with him. He was placed in a Title One reading program for kids behind in reading. He was taken out of class frequently for special teaching in anything they could. He was even in a special class to teach him to hold his pencil. Things were tough, and he was not making very good progress. The effects of the treatments that we chose for him were now hitting us in the face. We did talk to long term survivors and all of them said that learning and school were very difficult for them and had been a battle the whole time. This was not very encouraging for us or Nathan.

Then things started to turn around for Nathan. Not to say anything bad about his teacher at the time, but she went on maternity leave with eight weeks left to go in the school year. About three weeks later, we got a letter home saying that Nathan had been kicked out of Title One reading because he was now reading at grade level. He was now writing better because he had a new pencil grip that the substitute teacher found, and it worked much better for him. We started getting reports home that he was paying better attention and doing better overall. *What happened?!* I asked him. The simple truth is he did not work well with his previous teacher, and he worked great with his new teacher. The teachers had different styles. The new teacher was less strict, applying less pressure, and was supportive of any accomplishment. He flourished under her care. We were completely floored. Nathan had the answer the whole time and I did not ask him. Based on this experience, we started doing a couple new things. First: we include Nathan in all our discussions and plans for his education. He knows the approach we are trying, why we feel it will work, and what we expect him to do to help. He, in return, tries to the best of his ability. He lets us know if he thinks it is working and if he has any other suggestions. Second: before each school year, I sit down with his teacher and have a very detailed discussion on what they should expect. Gingerly, I let them know what Nathan needs from them to succeed. I stay very involved with the teacher throughout the year. In the good years, the teacher is a member of the team to get as much information in Nathan's brain that we can. This team approach has been very successful. The teacher knows I will back her decisions and discipline when Nathan acts out, and I know the teacher is giving him the extra attention he needs.

After completing first grade, we spent the summer trying to keep Nathan from losing any of what he learned in first grade. He read easy books and did dot-to-dot puzzles. We tried to point out, in the world, things that might be interesting. We were a lot more patient with him and that helped. That summer, the biggest help in his education was to relate the world to what he had learned in school. We would use his vocabulary words throughout the day. We would revisit any science lesson we could remember. The entire family went through first grade that summer.

When Nathan went to second grade, we were much more involved with the teacher. We now knew how important it was for Nathan to work well with his teacher. Nathan's second grade teacher was simply amazing with him. When we first met, we talked for about an hour getting to know each other and I tried to let her know what she was in for with Nathan over the next year. My first piece of advice for her was that he is not a faker. He does not lie, so if he is telling you he hurts or he is sore or he does not understand, please believe him. We started an excellent working partnership that evening. At one point in the conversation, I let her know when she needed to yell at Nathan, and was not going to, she could send a note home and I would yell at him for her. Her reply was, "*You are not allowed to yell at him either*". From that comment, I knew they would be an excellent pair. She was his tutor once a week after school. Nathan would miss a lot of school for treatment and illness; she would help him get caught up. That year Nathan made great progress. He was still not at grade level on all subjects and still needed extra help with some things, but he was getting closer and was starting to like school.

What I took away from these experiences was that Nathan was very smart. He still could remember anything that got into his brain; the problem was getting it through the "fog" and into his long term memory. We needed to find a way to bypass short term memory and get information directly into long term memory. I will not gloss over this; this is a very difficult task. Nathan and I have been working on it for a couple years now and are only now finally achieving some results for our efforts.

We have learned quite a few things that can apply to all kids with "chemo fog".

- They are not faking it. There really is a problem and I'm sure every child shows this in a different way.
- The teacher they have in school can make a huge difference. Nathan needed a less strict teacher that would bond with him and make school a good place to be. When Nathan had a stricter teacher, he was constantly trying to not get into trouble and not concentrating on learning. Each child has their own teaching style in which they thrive.
- It is important to have parental involvement with the teacher. You cannot simply send the child to school and expect them to learn. You and the teacher must work together trying out different teaching techniques, and both must carry through with them. The work a parent does at home is as important as the work done at school. If you show how important their schooling is to you by spending your time with your child, then they know how important it should be to them.
- The school can and will test your child if you request it. This testing should not be feared. It is not going to be a label your child gets stuck with; it is the mechanism the school uses to be able to get additional resources for your child. Yes, they will be considered special needs, but they are! They do need special attention to succeed. With the help available they can catch up to grade level and even excel. Without the extra attention, it may be very difficult.
- Schooling does not stop when they get off the bus or they have their homework done. Schooling is a nonstop event. The more things in their life that are related to the school work your child is doing, the better they remember it.

Nathan and I have tried many different "tricks" or techniques on each school subject to see which one helps him remember things. It is very important to find a way to try and "skip" the short term memory and go straight to long term memory. The best way we found to do this is to make learning really fun and exciting. That sounds easy enough, but truly is not. Below are some of the things that work for Nathan. I have broken them out by school subject.

Spelling

Nathan does not do well when he copies things over and over again. He hated to write, I'm sure his hand hurt, and he just could not handle copy spelling words three, five or ten times. We needed a new approach that would make him enjoy spelling words. One day I decided to make him laugh. Instead of writing his words a bunch of times he had to:

- Say the word
- Spell the word
- Say the word
- Make a funny sentence about mom or dad with the word
- Mom or dad would reply with a funny sentence with the word

With this one simple technique, his spelling tests went from the 50 percentile to the 100 percentile in one week. He still loves this, but now we all get involved in it. We all know what spelling words he has and we use them throughout the week in any way we can. We spend time together at the dinner table practicing them. You get extra "points' if you can use multiple spelling words in each sentence. We are all going to be better spellers soon.

Math

We have always assumed Nathan would take to math like both of his parents. Scott is a test pilot and I'm an aerospace engineer; we love math. Math is visual and intuitive to me. This is not the case for Nathan. Math, like spelling, requires a lot of repetitive memorization. Unfortunately, you cannot use the same techniques for math as you do for spelling. It is not like you can make up funny sentences about mom with math. You can however start counting by 2's or 3's or 5's. You can make up math problems out of everyday activities, you just have to change your mind set to do so. You have to make math fun and, for Nathan, it needs to be visual. The school had an online math game called FirstInMath that Nathan loved. He would get on the computer about 10 minutes a day and play with numbers. There are many other online games like this we go to on occasion to play. Flash cards work great if you can make them fun. Fun for Nathan is anything on mom's phone. So, my phone now has a flash card app on it for Nathan to play.

Reading

Reading was even tougher than spelling or math. Nathan hated it! I'm not even sure why he hated it so much. He just did. How do you make reading fun? We found a simple solution, audio books. Nathan would have his iPod on his head 24 hours a day if we let him. What is he listening to? Books. We started with the Magic Tree House books. We would listen to them in the car when driving to the hospital. He then memorized the Harry Potter books. I could only listen to each of the first five books about three times, and then I bought him a Walkman so he could listen to them without me. Recently, we added the Rick Riordan book series about Greek and Roman Gods. I have been told and agree that the next best thing to reading a book is to listen to a book. Eventually, we got him to read books more, 30 minutes of reading every day, no matter what. Again, we started with the Magic Tree House series of books. He knew most of these, so reading them was not a daunting task. With time he has come to love reading books as well as listening to them. It has taken years and lots of support, but we are finally getting him to be a book lover. We have learned, as with everything else, he retains more information from the books the more he enjoys them. He is now reading the Harry Potter books instead of listening to them and loving them.

Science

Science for us was a bit easier. Both Scott and I love to do science stuff. We have a general knowledge of all the science an elementary school child will learn and can help him with most things. The hardest part was to convince Nathan that we actually knew what we were talking about more than the boy next door that was Nathan's age. Apparently, the diplomas on the wall did not impress Nathan. We now run science experiments just for fun. Yesterday we were investigating condensation on the outside of a cup of ice water. We set up the experiment and then talked about what would happen to the cup when we got home. Nathan had missed the experiment during class so we just recreated it at home. For whatever science subject he is doing at school, we find a way to include it in our dinner conversation. We find that if we can connect whatever he is learning to an interesting story he does not forget it.

Social Studies

Nathan is studying Geography right now. He is learning the state names and where they are located. One week I had gone out of town for my 96 year old grandmother's funeral. I was not able to work with Nathan that week. He came home with a 20% on his geography test. This was confirmation that what we were doing was working. Now we needed to work on the Northeast states. Lucky for me I was raised there. The kids had vacationed at their grandparents' house in Massachusetts and on Cape Cod. We knew a lot of things about this area; we could make this fun. We went through all the states and told stories about them: what relative lived where, what vacation we took there, any exciting landmarks we knew of, anything that would get those state names into his brain. It worked. Two days later he took the same test and received a 100%. Go Nathan. This was our approach for the rest of the states. My son is lucky that we have lived in so many places over all our years in the Air Force and we can come up with funny stories about most states. Again, it is finding a way to make school work fun and entertaining so you can skip short term memory and get directly into long term memory. Any extra fun information helps get things to stick.

Behavior

Nathan had to learn how to act around other kids. He did not and does not understand what "personal space" is. He would be in other kid's faces, jump on their backs and generally be a pest. These areas required as much attention as the school work did. We could not blame Nathan; he had been under intense doctor's care for three years at the time. He had never had any privacy or personal space himself. But he was able to learn this too with the right threat of punishment. Nathan's favorite things to do was come home from school, get a snack and watch Pokémon for a half an hour, and then go and do his school work. If he could not behave properly in class, I would take TV away from him that afternoon. I had to implement this punishment once. Not jumping on a fellow student's back was now in long term memory. For Nathan, rewards always work better than punishments. As with everything else, behaviors are learned. We needed to set good examples and reward good behavior. When that did not work usually a very small "consequence" for his actions would translate into long term memory faster.

General Studying

It is hard for Nathan to remember a long set of instructions. The steps get jumbled up in his head and he cannot repeat it. We have found lists work very well. A great list example is sorting change. If you give Nathan a pile of money and tell him to count it, he does one coin at a time, 5 cents, 10 cents, 25 cents, 50 cents and so on. The change pile had over $30 of change in it. No matter how many times I told him to, *"Sort the coins, stack them in $1.00 piles and then count,"* he just did not get it. The solution was a short list of the steps. Then each time he practiced counting money he would read and follow the list. There was no pressure from me repeating over and over the instructions, he could just see them. Eventually, he just did it without the list.

Lists also helped him with math and other types of problems at school. The teacher let him tape this list to his table:

- Read the problem
- Do you understand what the problem is asking? If not, ask questions.
- Do you need help with anything? If you do, ask questions.
- Start the problem
- When you are looking around the room and not working, go back to step 1.

Humor works well with Nathan. Find your own methods that work with your child. They are out there, you and your child and their teachers just need to find them.

Muscle and Bone Pain

Nathan has had constant muscle and bone pain his entire journey. Leg pain and fever were the two symptoms that helped us find his disease. As treatments killed the cancer cells, his pain would increase. As treatments caused their side effects, his pain would increase. What was truly amazing about this pain was that Nathan's spirit never failed, his desire to ignore the pain and be like other little boys was his only desire in life.

Like many neuroblastoma children, Nathan had disease throughout his skeleton. Imagine small pockets of cancer in his bones. As the disease dies, holes are left behind in these bones, leaving gaps creating weakness until the bones heal. The main place in his bones for Nathan's disease was his right hip. It was the hottest spot on all the scans. With this large collection of tumor cells, Nathan's hip was compromised. The head of his femur was no longer round; this condition is called avascular necrosis. This is another common occurrence for neuroblastoma kids. Sometimes it heals and sometimes the kids just live with it. I have to believe, with all these skeletal and muscle issues that Nathan is in pain most of the time. Whenever he does any quantity of physical activity, he is in pain for days to follow. We only know this by watching him and observing his actions. He generally does not tell us he is in pain. This journey is tough on a small body.

With all the pain in their lives, we need to help them whenever we can. The pain is so prevalent in Nathan's motion. He just treats it as normal and continues whatever he was doing. We, as parents, need to set up the limits and guidelines for the children. I recommend meeting with the doctors and pain team to find the best medicines for your child. Don't hesitate to give them pain medicine when they show the very first signs of pain. It is very hard to catch up to pain with medicines once it has a hold on your child. Give them massages if they need them, hot baths, snuggling, anything that comforts them through it. Pain is something they should not need to fight through alone. There are medicines that can take pain away but still let them be kids. Our philosophy is to let him be a kid, let him run around and do what other little boys do, and then we treat the consequences as best we can. He cannot live in a bubble no matter how much we want to protect him. Besides, as I have described above, there would still be pain in the bubble. Even with these medicines and treatments, it is unlikely you will be able to remove all their pain. Unfortunately, this is just a fact of life for a cancer survivor. In the end, there should be a balance between pain and motion. Your child's action will be your guide.

Physical Therapy/Taekwondo

Physical Therapy (PT) needs to be present in your child's life on a continual basis from now on. It can be formal PT with a specialist or it can be other activities your child enjoys. My recommendation is to find an activity your child likes to do, a lot. It could be dance; it could be gymnastics. It could be anything, but find that one thing they love and let them do it. It is important they enjoy this activity MORE than they dislike the pain it causes.

After all of Nathan's treatment, he was very weak and physically unfit, but he was still here with us. He had a lot of trouble just walking. We were able to get him a wheel chair for longer excursions, but the day to day moving around was painful and our attempts to strengthen him physically was met with great resistance from him because it hurt so much. He had been given physical therapy in the hospital which helped him get stronger and heal faster, but, once we left the hospital, we needed to find something that would help him and that he was willing to do. We tried t-ball, but he hated being the slowest kid and did not want to go. We tried to work with him at home, but we were parents and always gave in when he hurt. Then we found Taekwondo. A friend of his had started a couple months earlier and loved it. We had the Master check him out and make sure it was safe. With the Master's agreement, we started Nathan in Taekwondo three times week. Initially, it was obvious to us that Nathan had some serious limitations to overcome. He could not lift his right leg very high, he could not balance at all, and he could not even run around the studio. Many nights after class he needed to have extra pain medicine so that he could function. Taekwondo was a big adjustment for him, but he kept going. He kept smiling and he kept trying each new skill as he was asked to do it. He got stronger and started to thrive. We had found the physical therapy that was going to work on Nathan.

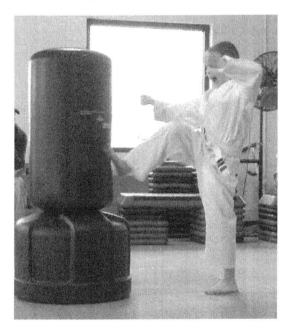

Figure 21 Nathan's Physical Therapy, Taekwondo

A friend of mine is a physical therapist for the children's hospital. She has seen the progress he had made with Taekwondo. She wanted to know how we got him to do all those things in class. She was having difficulty getting some other neuroblastoma kids to do their therapy. In the end, we agreed the most effective form of physical therapy was finding an activity Nathan liked so much he completely ignored the pain he was in. I want to give you an idea of how successful this has been for him. When Nathan started Taekwondo his right leg was very weak due to his avascular necrosis. It was rotated in towards his left leg and he could not lift his right foot above his left ankle. After a few months in Taekwondo, he could almost keep his right leg straight. A few months later, he could almost run. After three years he is a first degree black belt and can perform most of the moves just like any other black belt. He still has a little trouble with high kicks on his right leg, but he is amazing. Nathan still goes to three 45-minute Taekwondo sessions a week, and the instructors do not let him skip any of the activities. They are well aware of his physical issues and work through them, not around them. Now he is running around like any other boy his age and no one can tell what he has been through by observing his motions and actions. We, as his parents, always need to stay alert and pay attention. He is not like any other child, he does have certain things he cannot do or should not do. But as far as the other kids know, he is just like them.

Your child may not like Taekwondo. They may prefer dance, or baseball, or gymnastics. It does not really matter what the activity is as long as they love it and are willing to continue working at it. It is important the activity is two to three times a week and a lot of fun. Taekwondo has been so much fun for Nathan that the entire family started taking classes. The four of us are now first degree black belts and love it just as much as Nathan does.

Just Trying to be a Normal Kid

Nathan's overall driving force in his day to day life is to just be a normal kid like all the other normal kids. He wants to play sports; he wants to run around in the neighborhood. He wants to be a kid. We try to allow him to do this with certain restrictions. We try to limit these to only the necessary ones. For example, the chemotherapy has left his teeth with blunted roots. His teeth are not secure in his mouth the same way other kids are; therefore, we have asked him to not play tackle football in school or in the neighborhood and to wear a mouth guard whenever doing anything during which he might get hit in the jaw or face.

We try to help him with things that should come naturally but don't. For so long, Nathan has not been able to run with his toes pointing forward.

His hips and legs would not allow him to do it. It hurt when he ran and he ran very slowly. Over the past few years we have worked with him and actually had to teach him how to run properly with his toes pointed forward. His gym teacher at school even noticed his gate and helped him fix it. With extra attention, he now runs like most other little boys and is getting faster.

Our philosophy in Nathan's life for most things physical is to let him be a little boy and do the things little boys do and then deal with the consequences (e.g. pain and injuries). We feel we have been given extra time with him that we were not supposed to get since his disease was so severe. Therefore, we are trying our best to let him be, let him do those activities he wants to, and not smother him or put him in a bubble to protect him. Some days this is a lot harder than other days but that smile and those stories are worth it all.

NOTES

NOTES

CHAPTER 8. WISH TRIP

The Special Wish Foundation is one of many organizations that fulfill wishes for seriously ill children. Nathan was offered such a wish a few years ago. This section shows you what a trip like this is like. It is also our opportunity to tell some of the amazing stories about the people that treated us so well.

Nathan and Kate chose a trip to Orlando, Florida, for Nathan's wish trip. Nathan was given a week at Give Kids the World Village (see GKTW.org). It is a whole village designed for kids like Nathan and their siblings. Kids from the 70 different wish organizations in the U.S. visit them year round. You stay in the village in your own villa. They feed you, throw parties, and spoil your family for a whole week. The village has an arcade, dino putt putt, ice cream parlor, pizza place, theater, a carousel (which was Kate's favorite), and many other great activities for kids. When you are not in the village playing, you receive tickets to Disney, Sea World, and other Orlando attractions.

Our trip started when we were picked up by limousine on a Saturday morning. The kids were so excited they almost didn't change into their clothes and wanted to travel in their pajamas. We were met at each part of our trip by greeters and wonderful people to make Nathan and Kate feel like the most important people anywhere, ever. The kids loved flying on the airplane. They loved giggling at everyone and telling them they were going to Disney.

When we arrived at the village, we were shown the layout. It was a theme park on its own. They have a train, power boats, a carousel that Kate had us ride as often as she could, a pool and a water play area, just to mention a few. The Mayor of the village, Mayor Clayton (a rabbit), met us at lunch. He told us about the dancing and games. The kids settled right in and loved the place. There was a big bag of "stuff" for each of them when we got to our villa. The week continued like this with gifts, friends, and smiling people.

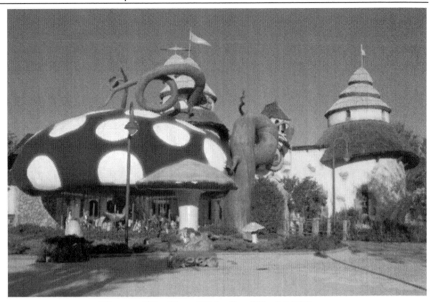

Figure 22 Give Kids the World Village

Our first full day was spent at Disney's Animal Kingdom. Animal Kingdom is Mom's favorite Disney Park and Mom was allowed to pick the first day. We climbed the dinosaurs, watched the tigers, took the safari ride, watched the 4-D Nemo in his own musical, and did the white water rapids ride, twice. The best part was watching Nathan on the rides. He did not understand that Disney is all "make believe" (except the animals, of course). When the bridge almost washed out on the safari ride, Nathan really thought the bridge was washing out. His face was priceless. Then Scott took him on the roller coaster where the Yeti was tearing the track apart. We did not tell him ahead of time it was fake (our bad). The poor guy was scared. He did not really trust us much after that. We did not mean to scare him, but his sweet face told a story. After the Yeti ride, we realized our mistake and let him know what Disney was and that he could be certain to enjoy the rides without worrying the Yeti was really going to attack him.

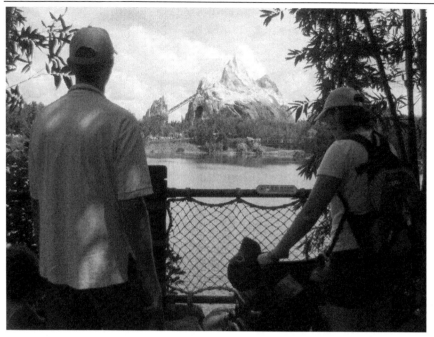

Figure 23 Eyeing the Yeti at Disney Animal Kingdom

The entire Disney organization was fabulous. They knew we were on a Wish Trip. They gave us passes that said, *"Do everything in your power to expedite this family to the ride."* They truly followed this philosophy. During our entire trip, Nathan was in a wheel chair and experiencing neuropathy in his hands and feet. Neuropathy is when your nerves swell and cause pain in your fingers and toes, which then moves up your arms and legs. He would not have done very well if he had to wait in lines and walk around. The staff and other visitors treated him and us very well.

The following day started with a visit from Mickey and Minnie Mouse at the village. For any big Mickey Mouse fans, you know that it is rare to see Mickey and Minnie together. In fact, they are never together at the Magic Kingdom; it is some kind of tradition. Kate LOVED seeing Minnie (the girl Mickey as she calls her). The kids hugged on them, had pictures taken, hugged some more. No one was in a rush; the kids were able to enjoy their time as long as they wanted.

We spent most of the day at the Wet-N-Wild water park. The kids complained constantly of the cold water, then jumped in. The park had big kid rides and little kid rides. Kate really had a blast in the water. This was a big step for her because before visiting this park she had been very scared to go in the water. This place was too much fun to not jump in. She even went down a really small slide a few times. When the nasty storm rolled in, we went back to the village to play with all the village stuff.

That evening was pizza movie night for Scott and the kids. GKTW Village has the best pizza and they bring it right to your villa. While the children were occupied, Grandma and I went shopping for souvenirs. One cannot go to Disney without getting a few souvenirs. Special Wish Foundation knew that; they even sent extra spending money for us. The kids were delighted when we got back. Kate had a new dress and would look like Tinker Bell the next few days. The Mickey and Minnie Mouse towels are still used every time they go to the beach. What a great exhausting day. Everyone slept very soundly that night.

We spent our third day at the Magic Kingdom. How does one describe the magic of two little kids in this wonderland? Kate had been waiting her three short years for this one day. She was finally going to see the princess castle. We had been talking about this for weeks and now it was here. After the ride over the water, we got to Main Street USA. I got ahead so I could see "The Face" when she finally saw it, and it was priceless. I didn't know if she was going to smile or cry. She did a bit of both. For the entire day, Kate was in her element. We spent our first hour at the castle: walking around the castle, looking at the castle, and making sure the castle was still there. Then we made it to fantasy land. We did the classics: Small World, Peter Pan, the Carousel, Mickey's Philharmonic (awesome show), and - did I mention - the castle. Kate did most of these in a haze. The bottom dropped out after getting to see the princess castle. She finally agreed to nap on my shoulder as we walked to lunch. She got about a 45 minute nap. I got a 45 minute snuggle. After, we were both our old selves again.

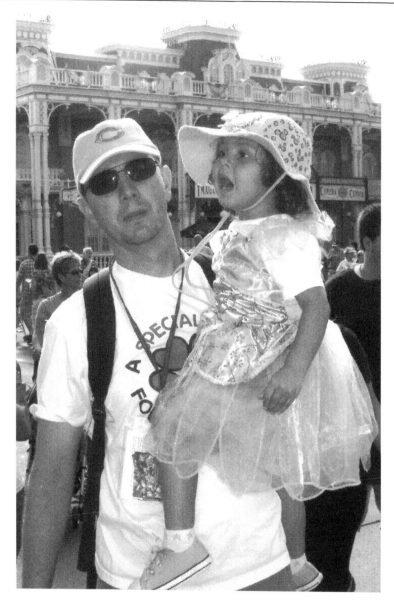

Figure 24 Kate's first view of the Princess Castle

Disney truly lived up to its name this day. We were once again escorted everywhere. In restaurants that had two hour waits, we were seated in minutes. The characters were brought to us since Nathan could not go to them. The kids had the most wonderful kid day. Disney will always be remembered by me for the way they treated my family on this trip. We all went home tired and happy and had the most restful sleep.

Day four was an easy, relaxing, play day at the village. The kids started with horseback riding. A local group brings in very gentle horses for the kids to ride. Both kids got to go twice around the track. The horses and the trainers took their time with the kids and horses. Kate was excited, then terrified, then triumphant on her ride. Nathan simply enjoyed the whole thing.

A little reality had to come into our visit. Nathan was still being treated and still needed to have medical stuff done. So, Scott and Nathan went to the local hospital to get labs drawn. The girls took this opportunity to visit the pool. This pool was great, the water was very warm and there were a lot of places for Kate to play.

Once the boys got back, we went on an air boat ride on the bayou. The air boat place had baby alligators that the kids got to watch while we waited. When the ride started, the boys (Scott and Nathan) started laughing and looking around and enjoying the air and the ride. Kate did not like this ride. I don't know if it was the noise, she had head phones on, or the boat, or the water or what, but it was the one thing all week that she did not want to do again.

That evening, the kids went to kid's night out. They played at the castle, had pizza, ate ice cream, and did a Village Idol. Village Idol is a lot like American Idol but for little kids. They get to sing or dance or do whatever they want. Our Nathan and Kate both got up to perform. Nathan sang the Pokémon theme song and Kate danced to it. The people at the Village said they did it in perfect unison and got a standing ovation. It was a very good down day for all.

The next day we spent at Sea World. As I said, I'm a big fan of how great Disney treated us. It is hard to say this, but Sea World treated us even better. Sea World people came up to us all day and escorted us to what they felt we needed to see. Nathan and Kate were greeted at the front gate and shown directly to where the Shamu character was hugging kids. They went up and hugged on Shamu, laughing and giggling.

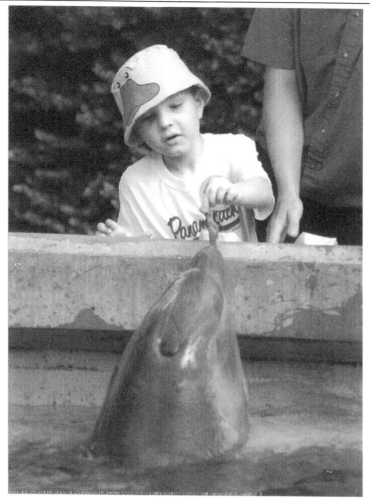

Figure 25 Feeding the Dolphins at Sea World

One of the highlights of Sea World was the dolphin feeding tank. Special Wish Foundation gave us tickets for Nathan to feed the dolphins a couple fish. That was not good enough for the Sea World staff. They let all of us feed the dolphins. The problem for the staff was the dolphins were just too far out of reach of the kids. The dolphin trainer saw this and had one of the dolphins jump on the ledge next to us. She, the dolphin, got her fish and jumped off. Nope, not long enough. Another dolphin came over up on the ledge and let all of us pet it. The day was the most memorable of the week.

Our last day was spent back at the Magic Kingdom. Kate got to see the princess castle again. Nathan got to drive the cars one more time. Scott got to ride Space Mountain. We all had one more ice cream cone. This is where our family tradition was started. If on vacation and you are asked if you want ice cream, the answer is always YES! Then we all got in the van, went back to the airport and flew home. The last treat of this magical week was the kids getting asked by the pilot if they wanted to visit the cockpit. Yup, they sure did.

These Wish Trips are truly a blessing. It gives the child a whole week of just being a child. There are no expectations on them. All they have to do is decide if they want ice cream or something else. Nathan's spirit was fully recovered from his very harsh treatments on this trip. He has never looked back.

NOTES

NOTES

CHAPTER 9. ORGANIZATIONS AND RESOURCES

Below are organizations we have had the pleasure to work with. There are many resources out there; please make use of them.

Children's Neuroblastoma Cancer Foundation

(CNCF)

CNCF is an organization of parents of kids with neuroblastoma. Their purpose is to educate other parents about this disease and then to fund research to cure it. I have been told that parents of neuroblastoma patients are a tight knit group and this organization is one of the reasons why. CNCF holds a parent conference each year where families and doctors come together to discuss the issues of neuroblastoma and how to solve them. Their website has a "Parent Handbook" that gives detailed information on everything you need to know about neuroblastoma. If you need help with anything, you can contact this organization directly.

Children's Neuroblastoma Cancer Foundation (CNCF)
360 W. Schick Rd., Suite 23 #211
Bloomingdale, IL 60108

Phone: (866) 671-2623
Fax: (630) 351-2462
Email: info@cncfhope.org
Website: http://www.cncfhope.org

Hospital Social Workers

Each hospital has a group of social workers available for the families. These people can help find the resources needed by a family, whether it is financial or something else. If you need anything outside of medical care at the hospital, ask for the social worker assigned to you.

Ronald McDonald House

The Ronald McDonald House is an organization with "houses" near hospitals. These Houses are available for families to stay in while caring for a sick child. The cost is minimal or free if money is an issue. Many local organizations bring in food and gifts for the children. It is a great option when getting treatment away from home or a good place to stay after bone marrow transplant or other long duration treatments. We stayed at two different Ronald McDonald Houses during our journey. One of them was for cancer patients only. We cannot say enough great things about this organization.

Ronald McDonald House Charities
One Kroc Drive
Oak Brook, IL 60523

Phone: (630) 623-7048
Fax: (630) 623-7488
Email: info@rmhc.org

Candlelighters

Candlelighters is an organization of parents at the local hospital level. This organization helped us with information and care at the hospital in which Nathan was diagnosed. They supported us with books they published to help with some of the major family concerns, for example other children dealing with a sibling with cancer, how to let the patient attend school, etc. Also the families that were in Candlelighters had a lot of local information on resources available at that hospital. Not all hospitals have a Candlelighters organization, so check where you are.

Livestrong

Livestrong is a foundation created to help people and families that are dealing with cancer. Their website has information on different types of cancer, how they can be treated and other resources available to help families find whatever they need. We used them to find an advocacy group to help address concerns with our insurance company. They were very professional and sympathetic to our situation.

LIVESTRONG
2201 E. Sixth Street
Austin, Texas 78702

Phone: (855) 220-7777
Website: http://www.livestrong.org/

Patient Advocate Foundation

Patient Advocate Foundation assisted us with discussing Phase I study insurance coverage for Nathan.

Patient Advocate Foundation Headquarters
421 Butler Farm Road
Hampton, VA 23666

Phone: (800) 532-5274
Fax: (757) 873-8999
Website: http://www.patientadvocate.org/

Corporate Angel Network

Corporate Angel Network is an organization that works with corporations that have commuter jets that fly regularly scheduled commuter flights. The corporation allows patients and their families fly on these jets for treatment. We were able to fly on The Limited's corporate jet many times to take Nathan to his antibody therapy. There was no cost to us and the crew on the airplane welcomed us with open arms. Nathan was able to visit the cockpit most flights.

Corporate Angel Network, Inc.
Westchester County Airport
One Loop Road
White Plains, NY 10604-1215

Phone: (914) 328-1313
Toll Free: (866) 328-1313
Fax: (914) 328-3938
Email: info@corpangelnetwork.org
Website: http://www.corpangelnetwork.org/

Project Angel Hugs

There are a few organizations out there just to make your child feel better just for a bit. Project Angle Hugs sends hugs to your child through the mail. These hugs come in the form of letters from other kids, cards, post cards, and packages of gifts. They are very thoughtful around most holidays, and they send a package of toys and gifts for your child. They even include presents for your other children, too. Nathan and Kate both squeal whenever they see an Angel Hugs box arrive in the mail. What a glorious few moments as they open it.

Project Angel Hugs
307 E. Mill Street, Suite 1
Plymouth, WI 53073
Phone: (920) 892-9138
Fax: (757) 873-8999
Website: http://www.projectangelhugs.com

Special Wish Foundation

Special Wish Foundation is one of the many organizations that fulfill the wish of a sick child. The wish can vary from a trip to Disney (like we took) to a play room (for a friend of ours) to a new computer for school. It just depends on the wish of the child and the ability of the organization to complete it.

A Special Wish Foundation, Inc.
National Headquarters
1250 Memory Lane N - Suite B
Columbus, Ohio 43209

Phone: (614) 258-3186
Toll Free: (800) 486-wish
Fax: (614) 258-3518
Website: http://www.spwish.org/

Give Kids the World Village (GKTW)

Give Kids the World Village is a resort in Orlando for sick children. GKTW works with the children "Wish" organizations to give children a week in the village. Its mission is to fulfill children's wishes and let them play like a child for a week. The village itself has enough things to do to keep anyone busy for a week. In addition they have tickets available for Disney, Sea World, water parks, alligator farms, air boat rides, etc. Our trip to GKTW is discussed in detail in the previous chapter. After you have been to GKTW for a wish trip, anytime you are in Orlando, you are welcome to go visit for the day. You can use their facilities, have a meal and play. We have been back once since our Wish trip.

Give Kids The World Village
210 South Bass Road
Kissimmee, FL 34746

Phone: (407) 396-1114
Toll Free: (800) 995-KIDS
Fax: (407) 396-1207
Website: http://www.gktw.org/

Children Oncology Group (COG)

The Children's Oncology Group (COG), is a National Cancer Institute supported clinical trials group. It is geared to childhood and adolescent cancer research. The COG has over 8,000 experts in childhood cancer at more than 200 children's hospitals, universities, and cancer centers across North America, Australia, New Zealand, and Europe. Many neuroblastoma trials are COG studies.

COG Group Chair's Office
The Children's Hospital of Philadelphia
3501 Civic Center Blvd, CTRB 10060
Philadelphia, PA 19104

Phone: (215) 590-6359
Fax: (757) 873-8999
Website: http://www.childrensoncologygroup.org/

New Approaches to Neuroblastoma Therapy (NANT)

The NANT consortium is a group of 14 Universities and Childrens Hospitals with strong research and treatment programs for neuroblastoma. Working together, they test new therapies for high-risk and relapsed neuroblastoma. NANT conducts clinical trials that test new drugs and new combinations of drugs against high-risk neuroblastoma. Those with promising results will then be considered for more extensive national testing.

NANT Operations Center
Childrens Hospital Los Angeles
4650 Sunset Boulevard, MS #54
Los Angeles, CA 90027-6016

Phone: (323) 361-5687
Fax: (323) 361-1803
Website: http://www.nant.org/

Neuroblastoma and Medulloblastoma Translational Research Consortium (NMTRC)

"The Neuroblastoma and Medulloblastoma Translational Research Consortium (NMTRC) is a group of 17 universities and children's hospitals headquartered at the Helen Devos Children's Hospital that offer a nationwide network of childhood cancer clinical trials. These trials are based on the research from a group of closely collaborating investigators who are linked with laboratory programs developing novel therapies for high-risk neuroblastoma and Medulloblastoma."

NMTRC
Helen Devos Children's Hospital
100 Michigan NE - MC 272
Grand Rapids, MI 49503

Phone: (616) 267-0335
Fax: (616) 391-2785
Website: http://nmtrc.org/

NOTES

NOTES

CHAPTER 10. FINAL COMMENTS

There are many, many, many organizations and people around to help you and your child. The number of loving, willing people astounds me. Let them help. Learn their stories. Help the next person.

We are forever changed by our journey through childhood cancer. We are all better people. We are truly blessed. We have been through this horrid disease, and we still have our son. It is my hope that our trials and experiences may help someone make their journey just that little bit easier.

CHAPTER 11. GLOSSARY AND ACRONYMS

ANC	Ratio of neutrophils to other white blood cells in the system. This ratio gives the doctors an idea of when your child is recovering from chemotherapy.
Antibody therapy	Immunotherapy where antibodies attach to neuroblastoma cells, the immune system then kills the foreign antibodies and the neuroblastoma cell attached to it
Avascular necrosis	Death to an area of bone due to lack of blood flow, can be a loss of roundness in a femur bone
Blood counts	Lab test that shows the levels of different blood cells and compounds in the blood stream, specifically hemoglobin, platelets, and ANC
Bone marrow biopsy and aspirations	Procedure where doctors put a hollow needle in the pelvic bone and take out a core sample of the bone marrow (soft part from inside the bone) and draw some blood from the bone that has bone marrow cells mixed in for testing
Bone marrow transplant	Intense chemotherapy to kill neuroblastoma that also destroys bone marrow, bone marrow needs to be restored by infusing patient's previously collected stem cells
Bone scan	Nuclear medicine scan that shows places of intense turn-over of the bone

Broviac catheter (central line)	A catheter in the big vessel of the heart for medication administration and blood draws.
Cancer	Bad guys
Chemotherapy	Single or cocktail of drugs designed to kill cancer cells
Cis Retinoic Acid	Immunotherapy oral drug that tells neuroblastoma cells to mature
Clear bone marrow	No cancer cells in the bone marrow
COG	Children's Oncology Group – A group of children's hospitals that facility research trials
Complete response	No evidence of disease after therapy
CT scan	Computed Tomography, slices of x-rays put together to create a 3-D image of your child, this scan allows the doctors to see in detail an area that may have disease or some other concern
Dose escalation	Drug doses are increased on a timeline to determine the highest safe dose
Frontline therapy	The best known therapy for a particular disease
Glomerular Filtration Rate (GFR)	Test to determine kidney function
Hematology	Study of blood disorders
Hem/Onc	Hematology/Oncology

Hemoglobin	Levels tell amount of hemoglobin (biologic substance that carries oxygen) in the red blood cells, low hemoglobin makes the child very tired and pale
Histology	Cellular level makeup of the tumor
Homovanillic Acid (HVA)	An acid found in your child's urine at small normal non cancer levels, neuroblastoma excrete the acid, giving an indication of the level of neuroblastoma activity, usually paired with VMA
IEP	Individual Education Plan
Individual Education Plan	A document that specifies the adaptations a child requires to be successful in school due to qualifying conditions as stipulated by law
Intravenous Immunoglobulin (IVIG)	Blood product from donors, rich in antibodies, that recognizes and helps fight certain infections
Metastatic disease	Cancer that has spread to multiple parts of the body from the primary tumor
MIBG	Metaiodobenzylguanidine – radioactive dye that is absorbed by neuroblastoma, one type is used for scanning, a different type and dose is used for therapy
MIBG Scan	Radioactive scan to test for neuroblastoma
MIBG therapy	Radioactive treatment for neuroblastoma, only available at a few hospitals

Minimal residual disease	Bulky tumors are gone, only a minimal amount of disease left
MRI	Detailed scan that uses magnets not radiation
Mucositis	Mouth sores – like canker sores in the mouth and throat, a painful side effect of chemotherapy
NANT	New Approaches to Neuroblastoma Therapy – group of universities and children's hospitals who research treatments for Neuroblastoma
Neuroblastoma	Bad guys
Neuropathy	An injury of the nerve endings that cause tingling in the hands and feet, severe neuropathy includes pain up the legs and arms.
Neutropenic	ANC that is below normal, patients are more susceptible to germs and catching bugs when neutropenic
Neutrophils	The white blood cells most critical to fighting germs
NMTRC	Neuroblastoma & Medulloblastoma Translational Research Consortium - group of universities and children's hospitals who research treatments for Neuroblastoma
No Evidence of Disease	Scans and tests show no evidence of any cancer
NPO	Nothing by mouth, no food or drink

Oncology	Study of cancer
Packed red blood cells	Blood product given when the hemoglobin is low
Paradoxical reaction	The exact opposite reaction to a drug than what is supposed to happen
Partial response	The drug removed a measurable amount of disease but not all of it
Petechia	Small blood extravasations into skin, looking like red spots, that may occur when the platelet levels drop below normal
Peripheral stem cell harvest	Procedure to take stem cells out of the blood to be used later to recover from bone marrow transplant
Platelets	Part of the blood system that allows the blood to clot, if the platelets are low patients may bleed or bruise easily
Port-a-cath (called "port" for short)	A type of central line that stays under the skin, the port is accessed with a needle
Primary tumor	The place the cancer started, for neuroblastoma, it is commonly on an adrenal gland
Progression	When the disease gets larger or more extensive instead of smaller
Radiation therapy	Radiation to primary tumor bed and other areas of concern
Remission	When cancer is completely eradicated by treatment and stays away

Stage of disease	A way for doctors to classify cancers and determine appropriate treatment
Toxicity	Severe side effects
Transfusion	When a blood product is given into the vein
Treatment protocol	Specific sequence of medications and test used for particular disease therapy.
Vanillylmandelic Acid (VMA)	An acid found in your child's urine at small normal non cancer levels, neuroblastoma excrete the acid giving an indication of the level of Neuroblastoma activity, usually paired with HVA

NOTES

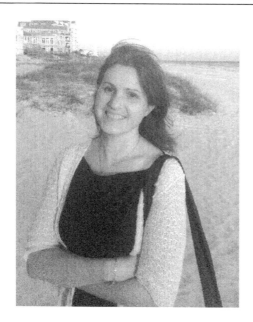

Rachel Ormsby is a wife, mother of two and aerospace engineer. When not running a household, she develops science hardware for the space program. This has included experiments on the Space Shuttle looking for new treatments for cancer, a cure for deafness and new ways to treat bone disease. Most recently she has worked on a bone densitometer for the International Space Station. She is the author of many scientific publications and co-holder of a patent. Rachel is the mother of Nathan and Kate. Nathan was diagnosed with Stage IV Neuroblastoma in August of 2006 when he was three and Kate was just one year old. When Nathan was diagnosed, she extended a planned "maternity leave" from her engineering career by an additional 7 years to care for Nathan and Kate. She has been married to her husband, Scott, since 1992.

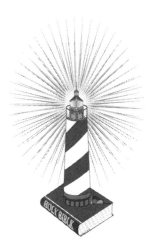

MJ Ministries Inc. was founded in January 2010 by Rev. Mamie Johnson. Growing up in less than desirable circumstances, her ability to develop and thrive was significantly compromised. It was through the love and compassion shown by strangers that she was able to overcome many obstacles. It is with that backdrop, Rev. Johnson formed MJ Ministries Inc. MJ Ministries seeks to convey the message of God's all-encompassing love through the concept of L.I.V.E. (Love, Integrity, Vision, and Empowerment). John 10:10 (King James Version) tells us *"The thief cometh not, but for to steal, and to kill, and to destroy: I am come that they might have life, and that they might have it more abundantly."* As God's love is received, all are encouraged to share that love with others.

As a people, we are faced with many obstacles but God has a way of making these obstacles bearable by way of His Son whom He gave as a sacrifice so that we could live.

MJ Ministries promotes the concept of L.I.V.E. by helping others through varying facets of life. It is also the goal of MJ Ministries to aid all people in realizing their potential and to pursue it. With the help of skilled volunteers, advisors, and the financial support of selfless givers and grants, we are able to provide direction, resources, counseling, and workshops to help others in their life challenges. We recognize that one size does not fit all but we believe sincere love can have a significantly positive impact on the world. We look forward to hearing from individuals with spiritual needs, providing support and direction.

Rev. Johnson, a licensed and ordained minister of the gospel, holds a Bachelor of Science degree in Business Management from the University of Phoenix and a Master of Arts degree in Theology from Xavier University in Cincinnati, Ohio. She is also the author of "When God Doesn't Stop the Rain (an autobiographical account of the many adversities she faced, and how accepting God's love helped her overcome them. The book is available at www.amazon.com). Along with serving as President of MJ Ministries Inc., Rev. Johnson serves as an Assistant Pastor and as a facilitator and speaker for many ecumenical initiatives.

MJ Ministries, Inc.| P.O. Box 498999 | Cincinnati, OH 45249
MJ Ministries, Incorporated © 2010
mjministriesinc@gmail.com
MJ Ministries Inc is a qualified IRS Section 501(c) (3) Organization

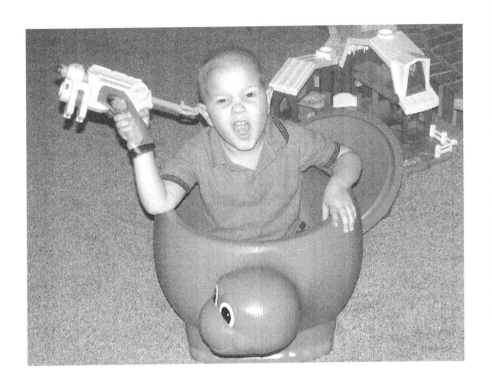

32688373R00114

Made in the USA
Charleston, SC
24 August 2014